Precious Lives Painful Choices

A prenatal decision-making guide

Sherokee Ilse

With special contributions by

Judith L. Benkendorf, M.S.
Susan Erling
Sheila Maland
Lara Palincsar
Carol Randolph

Edited by
Carol Frick

ACKNOWLEDGMENTS

Many people, parents and professionals alike, have shared their stories, expertise, regrets, suggestions and thoughts with me during the writing of this book.

I am deeply grateful to those who spent hours offering their experience, expertise, ideas and editing assistance: Judith L. Benkendorf, M.S., genetic counselor, Georgetown University Medical Center; Lara Palincsar, M.S., genetic counselor, Georgetown University Child Development Center and Sheila Maland, a mom and support group leader for these special families, who is working on her Masters in Counseling Psychology. My editor, Carol Frick, and my colleagues Susan Erling Martinez and Carol L. Randolph helped tremendously in their supportive and meticulous ways.

Also a special thanks to each of the parents, nurses, clergy, physicians, social workers and genetic counselors, many who remain unnamed and those listed below who shared their ideas and perspectives:

Faye Bailey, Shari Baldinger, Judith Calica, Joette Cates, Deborah Davis, Ph.D., Maribeth Wilder Doerr, Bob Fluck, Suzanne Fluck, Judy Friedrichs, Darlene Gibson, Susan Gordon, Gwen Griffin, Dr. Susan Hodge, Mary Johnson, Dorothy Kavanaugh, Shelley Kroeger, Lynn Kuba, Russell Kuba, Mary Kuehnl, Annalise LaHood, Jackie Minich, Monica Nelson, Tim Nelson, Thomas L. Pinckert, M.D., Debra Ramsey, Casey Reiser, Barb Schaak, Susan J. Scott, Rev. Rebecca Sherwood, Joellen Taylor, and Wendy Uhlmann.

9 8 7 6 5 4 3   Printed in the United States of America
Cover design: Bob Wasiluk and Tim Nelson, deRuyter Nelson Publications
Printing: Lakeland Press
Copyright 1993 by Sherokee Ilse.   Revised 1995.

For additional copies write to:
   Wintergreen Press
   3630 Eileen Street
   Maple Plain, MN 55359
   (612) 476-1303

New Area Code 952

Price $9.95/Bulk rate available for multiple copies.   ISBN 0-9609456-9-5

Precious Lives Painful Choices

A Prenatal Decision-Making Guide

To my loving husband, David,
and our children, Trevor and Kellan,
who fill our days with life and laughter,
and Marama, Brennan and Bryna,
who will always live on in our hearts and memories.

And in honor of all the special babies, those who live and those who have died. Among them: Stacey Danielle Bailey, Noah Cates, Laura Spring Fluck, Jenna Griffin, Lisa Ann Kaminski, Baby Kroeger, Francis Edward LaHood, Davon William Johnson, Riley Joyce, Alyson Kuba, Garrett, Christina Ramsey, Meghan Rose Maland, Michael John Minich, Margaret Mullenmaster Nelson and Matthew Michael.Scott.

THIS BOOK IS FOR YOU if you have a decision to make during pregnancy because you have received abnormal or unusual prenatal test results. If you are pregnant with multiple babies and are considering selective reduction, if you are considering carrying the pregnancy to term, giving the baby up for adoption or ending the pregnancy, the material presented will relate to you.

TO USE THIS BOOK notice that it is divided into many sections so you can immediately identify the topics that meet your needs. Because the sections were written to respond to the breadth of parental concerns at the appropriate time of need, you will notice that information is repeated in several sections if you read the book straight through. You may find different sections of this book helpful at different times. Other parts won't apply to you at all. It is very appropriate that you seek out sections, paragraphs and resources that deal with your situation and are helpful to you. Even if you use only two pages and that helps you clarify and make a better decision, I will consider this project a success. Use what you want to and let the rest go. The **Table of Contents** and the **Index** will help you locate what you need.

Two sections, **Continuing the Pregnancy** and **Terminating the Pregnancy**, present many aspects of each choice. Quotes, testimonials from parents, and suggestions about what kinds of experiences each choice might bring are included throughout the text. There are a number of other sections that may be helpful when the time is right. The **Appendix** presents resources for each situation.

You will notice this book is written to one reader. Whether you have a partner or are single, the book attempts to speak to you, the one reading it at the time. You may also note that due to the many procedures and physical needs at this time, many things are addressed to the mother, though it will not always specifically state this. Fathers are invited and encouraged to feel included in these pages and to recognize the many facets of this important process in which the father and mother are equally affected. Since few men have shared their comments openly with me, it was difficult to find quotes from many men. In order to add a stronger male perspective in future revisions, male readers are encouraged to send in their stories and share their needs and feelings.

CONTENTS

In memory of all those special babies
whose parents I have had the privilege of caring for—

Child,
Stay in my heart,
Where I will carry you with me
Forever.

Judith L. Benkendorf, 1993

PREFACE

My first book, *Empty Arms*, was written for those who have unexpectedly had a child die before, during or after birth. From the thousands of readers who have contacted me since the publication of that book, I have learned that there can be other agonizing aspects to pregnancy which are not being addressed at this time. While I am aware of the swirling public controversy and confusion that exist, my heart aches for families who find themselves in the position of having to decide, under great pressure and with little guidance available, the fate of their baby during pregnancy. With this new book, I seek to aid these special families as they search for the choice that best fits their hearts.

The goal of this book, *Precious Lives, Painful Choices*, is to provide a sensitive, comprehensive and balanced picture of the options available to you if you find yourself in the difficult position of having to decide the course of your pregnancy which has been shown to have serious problems. It is not intended to tell you what to do. Its purpose is to provide needed information, to help you ask questions you might not otherwise think of, to allow you to share in the stories of others who have been in similar circumstances, to offer a long-term perspective, and most of all to offer you nonjudgmental guidance and support.

When there is an abnormal prenatal diagnosis, it is common to be unprepared about what to do next. Most people I talk with state that they are given good medical care, but many do not know where to find information or even what questions to ask themselves or the medical community as they seek to understand their options. Even those who prepare themselves to make a particular choice if testing reveals problems need support to continue with the plans they have made.

Many people admit feeling pressured by family, their conscience, or the medical community to terminate the pregnancy, get on with healing, and look ahead to trying for another baby. Others share the pressures they feel not to consider termination because their family, their caregivers, others or they themselves strongly believe that abortion, even under such circumstances, is wrong. Still others experience support or pressure to end the pregnancy, yet their medical caregivers send them a confusing and painful message when they refer them to an abortion center or another facility for the procedure. Many people find it hard to get support for the decision they finally make. They feel undermined

1

and intensely pressured. Yet, there is another group of people who feel truly supported in the decision they choose.

Decisions such as these present a highly stressful situation, made more confusing and hurtful by the emotions of the abortion debate and the rules and regulations that further complicate a sad and unexpected experience. This can become a life-altering dilemma. The baby may have problems such as Down syndorme, spina bifida or disabilities of varying severity. The baby's problems might appear to be lethal: if the baby makes it to delivery she or he may not live long. Multiple babies may make selective reduction a necessary consideration in an effort to give at least some of the babies a better chance to live. Maybe adoption of the baby is a consideration.

Families are often expected to make a choice if there is a serious problem in their pregnancy. Well-informed and empowered parents can and will make careful and conscientious decisions based on their own needs, values and beliefs as they contemplate their future.

This book will present passionate pleas and stories for termination *and* for non-intervention in which parents either kept the baby or gave him or her up for adoption. Selective reduction experiences will also be presented by parents who have *been there*. Regrets and feelings of thankfulness will ring out. This is not to sway you toward one decision or the other, but to invite you to understand that each choice is full of passion, possible regrets, pain, love, and maybe even joy and beauty, eventually. Each choice will present a challenging journey that will likely involve deep grieving as you move toward healing.

I am so sorry that you are forced to be on this journey. There are no shortcuts or easy paths to take. The road is often difficult and lonely. Yet, I believe you can make it, and perhaps even grow wiser and stronger because of it, in time. Try to be positive and cautious as you go forward to face the struggles ahead. Be thoughtful, seek guidance and look within yourself. As hard and unfair as this situation seems, only you will be able to make this painful choice. In spite of the time pressures you may face, if you make your decision thoughtfully now, in the future you will be able to look back and say, "I made the best decision I could have at the time."

With love,

Sherokee

Sherokee

INTRODUCTION

"As a parent my role has been life-giving, not life-ending. Now I am in a dilemma of the greatest magnitude." A parent

"Prenatal tests are opening a window into the womb. Parents are having to answer some of the toughest questions life can ask.." (Granat 1991)

Prenatal testing, now a routine part of pregnancy, brings information that parents often want, and medical caregivers are eager to give. The fear of such problems as Down syndrome, spina bifida, sickle cell anemia, heart problems, Tay-Sachs disease, cystic fibrosis or other birth defects motivates caregivers and prospective parents to pursue or agree to available testing. Parents hope for reassurance that their baby is healthy. Sometimes the knowledge resulting from prenatal tests adds to the burden of anxiety. Little can be done when parents learn there is something wrong with the baby. Few *in utero* therapies currently exist to correct the problems, therefore the information does little to change the circumstances or cure the baby.

The question of "What will we do if something is wrong with the baby?" is difficult even to contemplate. For many the answer may be somewhat obvious, in theory. In actuality, however, abnormal test results present a decision parents are rarely fully prepared to make. Parents may find themselves going against their original hypothetical decision, sometimes even against their own beliefs. Some resist bonding with their baby while they wait for the test results, trying to lessen the pain of the decision they have already made.

"After watching our baby slowly die over his first two years of life from Tay-Sachs disease, we definitely decided we would have prenatal testing. That is the only way we dared to attempt another pregnancy." Anna

"We had selective reduction at 10 weeks from four embryos to two. I loved those babies and always will. We made our painful decision after many agonizing discussions with several doctors about the high odds of losing them all and possibly my life also. Being Christians and believing life begins at conception, we found this to be a tremendous decision. We were trying desperately to give our children the best possible chance of surviving." Angie

3

"No matter what the tests said, I do not believe in abortion and I could not have ended my baby's life. While we struggled with the news, we accepted that we would continue with the pregnancy." L.

Today's growing technology leads us to places we might never have imagined. Testing during pregnancy, such as ultrasound, maternal serum alpha-fetoprotein (MSAFP) screening and now the newer triple screen, and amniocentesis and chorionic villus sampling(CVS), is commonplace. Though most test results are normal, when there is an abnormality your entire family is naturally disrupted and distraught. You are required to make a choice. Even if you started the pregnancy knowing there might be a risk you may, like others, find yourself examining the difference between life and quality of life. If death of the baby is inevitable you may wonder if death now, by your decision, or a natural, non-intervention approach is better.

Previous generations have not faced this dilemma. Problems with the baby were usually not detected until *after* birth. The new parents had few decisions to make. Their coping and grieving began after the shock subsided. This is not so in most cases today. Now, the news often comes early and unexpectedly, and with it the power to decide whether or not to end this baby's life. The shock is still there and the grief still comes, along with the pressure and the responsibility of having to decide your child's fate.

The process of loving, hoping, dreaming, letting go and mourning is much the same as that which follows miscarriage, stillbirth, infant death, or living with a child with disabilities, but with added complications. Some of the added burdens are: choice, going through a termination or birth procedure, the societal pressures and response to each choice, and the very intense, potentially destructive feelings of *responsibility* and possibly *guilt* for ending a life and for choosing the timing and method of ending that life. A sense of failure for producing an imperfect baby, passing down "imperfect" genes or somehow creating problems in your baby may add to the already intense feelings.

GETTING THE NEWS—
SHATTERED DREAMS

"We lost all our dreams. We spent years planning and dreaming about playing catch in the yard and Little League. Then all of a sudden, boom, they're gone. When you get bad news it is earth shattering." Don

A precious pregnancy began, and with it your hopes and dreams intensified. These dreams, hopes and plans for your baby are real, whether now isn't the right time or you have wanted a baby for a long time. There are years of emotional investment in every child conceived. Bonding and preparation for parenthood begin in the parents' own childhood and continue to build throughout life. Those dreams are shattered and your plans are seriously altered when a problem is revealed during a pregnancy or shortly after a birth.

When you learned you were pregnant and underwent testing you probably felt optimistic that you wouldn't need to think through the "what will we do if..." You were seeking reassurance or just expecting a normal, healthy pregnancy and baby. Or maybe you had the testing done because you were worried there might be something wrong and you have been waiting for the results before you "get invested in this baby." Maybe you were not even sure if you wanted this baby in the first place.

You have just been given devastating news; maybe something suspicious was diagnosed during a routine check-up or ultrasound examination. Maybe you have been going through prenatal testing or a series of tests and a problem was found. There is something wrong with your baby, your pregnancy or possibly even with you, the mother. Maybe the baby has an abnormality which will affect the quality of life. It might be life threatening, a major problem or a less severe defect. You may have twins, one with a problem and the worry about what will happen to the healthy one. Maybe you are carrying many babies, too many for a safe delivery, you fear. A nightmare has begun—one that requires a decision.

What will you do? You face a difficult choice. Even *no* decision is a decision. Should you end the pregnancy or let it proceed? The fear of either can feel overwhelming. These things happen to other people,

5

not to you! This situation feels awful and you have a right to whatever feelings you are now experiencing, no matter how overwhelmed and shocked you must feel. You may be wishing the problem would go away. Perhaps you wish that nature would take care of the problem for you. You may ask yourself if this could be a mistake, if the test results could be wrong. Do not let these concerns and feelings paralyze you.

"I wished that nature would take care of this for me. Sometimes I hoped for a miscarriage. That was something I didn't have any control over, so I wouldn't be faced with the decision." Amy

"I was not convinced that a fourth baby was a good idea in the first place. When the problems were found there was anger at everyone and everything, including at Monica. I fought the feelings of 'I told you so,' because I knew how destructive this could be. Ultimately I needed to realize that I had been as responsible for this pregnancy as she and we must face together whatever the future would bring." Tim

Unfortunately, this *really is happening* and now you need critical information quickly. But how do you do this in the middle of a crisis with so little experience and knowledge of the choices and the long-term consequences? To further complicate the situation, you probably have been told there is little time to decide. There is no perfect solution. It might seem like choosing between the unthinkable and the unbearable. You are being asked to decide whether you can raise a handicapped child or carry a dying baby to term, yet you may not be sure of the severity of the problem. It may be anguishing to have to even consider the idea of aborting your loved baby. Your wanted baby may now turn into an unwanted baby. To end the pregnancy or to continue, to choose to end the life of some babies hoping the others will live—each decision brings challenges, risks and problems. Every option comes with pain. A sense of failure may consume you. Ambivalence and guilt may confuse you.

"I didn't feel guilty for having thought that termination was a possibility. I could only consider alternatives based on information I was receiving." Tim

You will need guidance and support in making the best decision you can. Do not allow others to persuade you into choices that you don't wish to make or are not ready to make. Your physician, a clergyperson, geneticists, co-workers, counselors and friends cannot tell you what to do, even though you may be tempted to seek an answer from them or they may offer answers. While some will share thoughts of what they might do if in your shoes, they are not you and they cannot decide for you. These individuals can help you gather information and guide you in determining the most helpful questions to ask. Be sure to do what you feel *you* need to do and what *you* can live with, not something that is another person's idea of what is best for you. The personal choices you make will affect you from today on.

Why did this have to happen to me, to us?

You have every right to question why this has happened. You don't deserve it and it seems unfair. You may cry out, "Why, God?" or "Why me?" You may have really wanted this baby for a long time, and perhaps it has even taken you some time to conceive. Maybe your pregnancy was unplanned and came as a surprise. Or maybe this was not a wanted baby, especially at first. You might feel guilty. In your thoughts you might go over and over every aspect of your pregnancy searching for something you did that could have caused this problem or for something you could have done to prevent it. You might feel as though you are being punished because of such thoughts or for some past deeds. You might blame yourself or your partner, even though logically you know your reaction is unrealistic. You may hope this nightmare will end and that you will wake up to find that everything is back to normal. All of these feelings and reactions are normal. In fact, most people go through some of this thinking in the early hours and days of their crisis. Asking "Why?" is a common cry of pain. An answer is not likely to come. Let your "whys" come and share them with others.

"After three miscarriages and two years of infertility I remember exclaiming, 'Why? I thought I paid my dues!' What more could I possibly deal with? How could I be asked to consider terminating a baby I wanted so badly and fought so hard for?" Lynn

IMMEDIATE CONCERNS

"Your baby (or pregnancy) has serious problems." Such powerful words! These words might now echo in your head along with your many questions, concerns and fears. The time between hearing this devastating news and having to make a decision is usually short. This is a time in life where there is no compromise and no middle ground. A decision must be made.

Though the choices sound simple in words—**ending the baby's life now, or letting nature take its course then either keeping the baby or giving him/her up for adoption**—all are quite complicated in reality. For some people, being pregnant with multiple babies brings up the question of **selective reduction.**

If you decide to interrupt the pregnancy and the baby is still alive, or if you need to consider whether you will have a reduction of some of the babies you are carrying, there are legal time limits that vary from state to state after which termination is no longer an option. This makes a careful, well thought out decision difficult. You need time to think this through. *If you do need extra time now, try to slow things down if at all possible.*

Resist the urge to make a quick decision. The feelings of hopelessness and of being rushed may be hard to shake. Give yourself the time you need to research the options, facts, and medical information, as well as to explore your emotions, beliefs and values. Look within yourself to find the direction. This might be accomplished in quiet contemplation, prayer or meditation. Make time for yourself now. You may want to take a few days off work to gather the information and your thoughts to make a plan. In addition, find a supportive relative, friend or care provider.

You might think that if you choose one option, such as abortion, that it will be a shortcut, an ending, a chance to make the decision and then put it behind you. Maybe you are inclined to make a quick decision to continue the pregnancy because it is too difficult to deal with the reality of the baby's condition, or it is too hard to wrestle with your conscience. You shouldn't expect a quick fix or an easy escape. When a baby dies, no matter how or when, or when a baby lives, but with problems, there is pain, anguish and sorrow. When the parent is the one to decide the timing of this death, overwhelming feelings of

8

sadness, remorse and often guilt may follow. You may start to grieve even before you are aware of feeling grief. Anger and other feelings will surface as part of the grieving process.

It is important to realize that there is no one right answer for everyone. Your options might be limited by your situation, but weigh the options you *do* have carefully. While termination may be the right answer for some, continuing the pregnancy will be right for others. Reduction of some of the babies may be an option for you, or it may not be. Ultimately it will be you who must live with the consequences of your decision. What's in your heart is most important. Use your internal and external resources—your spirituality and your support system—to reach your decision. In many ways the choice you make will represent not an ending—a final solution—but the first steps down a path which will lead you through pain and heartache. You will face unexpected challenges and changes, but eventually you may feel peace, acceptance and recognize that you have grown.

"I felt the decision I needed to make was the ultimate in motherhood, in parenthood, in responsibility for a child who was uniquely my own. There is great fear, but also strength in this. After all, no one had the right to make this decision but me. No one had the right to the pain or the love, but me. I cried and embraced both." Carol

"While I sometimes think about what it would be like to have four children, I don't look upon my decision with regret or remorse. We made the best decision we could at the time, based on many issues and feelings. We have a wonderful family, filled with love and happiness." Susan

One of the most important things to remember is that your baby is loved; believe that your baby feels that love coming from you. Whatever you decide, do it out of love for your precious child.

"It didn't seem like love, though, when everyone was just talking medical facts. It sometimes felt very cold, logical and unfeeling. It was hard for me to accept that I made such a logical, rational decision about my own child. At times I didn't feel like a loving mother." Debra

"I believed in my heart that my baby felt all my love. As I struggled to decide I kept this in my mind and it helped me." S.

"Being an engineer, I'm the logical type. The advice from some of the doctors to terminate the pregnancy seemed so practical and rational, when you only considered the facts and statistics. However, that

9

ignored all the important factors like values, morals, emotions and love. This presented a major conflict for me, since the logical side of me heard the statistics and sought the 'practical' answer. But in the end I knew the other factors had to be given strong consideration; they would be what I had to live with every day." Bob

I feel numb and in shock. Am I grieving?

Shock, numbness, confusion and fear are all common grief responses in the early hours and days after receiving such overwhelming news. Feelings of craziness are not unsual. You may walk around in a fog, easily confused, with many moments of sadness, anger and despair. These are but some of the early rush of feelings. Disbelief is typical, along with second thoughts about why you ever had the testing done in the first place. Your previous intellectual decision about what you would do if the tests came back with abnormal results may seem foreign to you. You might have to remake the decision *emotionally* now because the reality of the situation, with all its far-reaching implications, is more complex and personal. You may even feel like a different person.

"I remember after they told me there was a sac at the base of my baby's skull I thought, They're wrong, I know this baby is fine. The ultrasound tech then asked me if I wanted the pictures. I burst into tears and pushed them away, not knowing if I should bond with the baby or not." Lynn

"There is no joy in this pregnancy now, only fear...I was preparing for a real birth, not a death." Barbara

"Before I found out that our baby had problems, I felt beautiful and full of life. After the test results, I felt horribly ugly and couldn't stand to look at myself in the mirror. I even felt dirty. I wanted to have it all over with." A.

Feelings of "worthlessness" or "ugliness" may surface but they eventually disappear. It is not "all over" when the baby is no longer inside you. In many respects, the grieving-healing process is just starting. You are beginning a new stage of your life without that healthy, wished for child, but with a heightened sense of vulnerability. You fear that you might never experience another worry-free pregnancy again because you know that the worst can happen...it seems it has.

You are probably already grieving as you contemplate your decision. This surely was not in your plans. Anger and other feelings are a

10

necessary component of the grieving process. If you are somewhat prepared for the possible responses it might be a little easier to handle. Reading and talking with others can help you begin to understand grief and the process of mourning.

Where do I begin?

Becoming educated and examining your beliefs and needs are critical at this point. You might have time constraints to take into account if termination is an option you are considering. The longer you wait, the more likely that laws about termination will dictate your decision. In some cases, gestational age will determine methods of termination. The following suggestions may help you to gather information and move forward. You decide which are useful in your decision-making process:

Be as certain as you can about the diagnosis. Talk about reliability, further tests, other expert opinions, statistics, and what the literature and studies say about this problem. This will be discussed in more detail later. This is the important logical/factual side of making the decision.

Seek as much information as you can handle. Find not only medical information, but also learn about the possible emotional and spiritual effects a decision can have on you and your family. Use this book's **Appendix**, a public, medical or church library as well as other support organizations. Although it may be hard to ask for help, this will be important. Your medical team may be able to provide you with names of organizations that deal with your baby's problem or abnormality. Read and talk with others to get this information. Find out what resources might be available to you and your child in your area. You might benefit from a support group, and emotional and spiritual counseling. Learn about the doctrines of your religion with regard to termination. The position of your church may be a strong factor in your decision. One couple in Australia was excommunicated from their church after they terminated their pregnancy. They realized too late that they had not thought to investigate this before they made their decision. Whatever your concerns are, ask for help in getting what you need or want.

Talk with others who have faced similar situations. Unless you know people who have faced a similar situation, it might be hard to find someone to talk with who really understands. The fear of being stigmatized keeps some people from freely discussing this personal issue with others. You can ask your medical caregiver, a genetic counselor, or use the resource list in the **Appendix** to help you find support organizations or individuals who have had similar circumstances. Once you have found someone, ask about their reasons for continuing or interrupting their pregnancy. How has their decision affected their lives? If their child is alive, what is his/her life like? Would they make the same choice again? If the parents ended the pregnancy, or aborted some of the babies, how did they share their loss with others? If they had to do it over again, would they still make the same decision? If no, why not? If yes, how could the situation have been improved? There are a few books out now that also explore these areas.

"Through Pen Parents, a support network, I was connected with a person whose situation was almost identical to mine. I wrote to her and we have begun corresponding on a regular basis. I see a long and wonderful friendship developing between us. I am thankful to have found this support." Shelley

"We spent hours talking with parents of quadruplets and twins, learning about high risk pregnancies and the financial burden of a large family. Our most basic questions could not be answered. No one could tell me what type of pregnancy I would have and what the future would bring us." Susan

Build a support system. You may want to discuss your situation with people close to you besides your partner. While this may not be easy, you may want to find someone, a relative or friend, who has previously been supportive and whom you trust. They might be able to see aspects in this dilemma that you hadn't thought of. They might know someone who has had a similar experience. You may want to share your problem with at least a few people who care about you. A decision of this magnitude is a difficult burden to bear mostly alone. If you have a clergyperson or pastoral counselor in your life this might be a good time to turn to them for assistance.

"During the decision-making process, we spoke to only a couple of friends about having to make this decision. I didn't want people's opinions of what they would do, even if they agreed with me. I wanted to surround myself only with professional people who could give me facts about either option, without inserting their personal bias." Gwen

Explore the potential impact on your family and your baby. You may want to consider your family's needs and the needs of the baby. What are the possible risks and benefits with each choice? If the baby has severe problems but will most likely live, you may find yourself thinking about quality of life issues versus life itself. You may ask yourself: How much will the baby suffer? Will the baby be born alive? How long will treatment likely go on? How would I care for a critically ill baby? How might my physical health be affected? What might the emotional impact be on me if I continue to carry the pregnancy? or end it? What are the financial implications? If the baby is likely to die sometime during pregnancy or after birth what are my options? How will the baby die? Will non-intervention give me enough time to learn and prepare for what is to come? Will it be better to keep the baby alive *in utero* for as long as possible? Or out of concern, will I want to make the decision soon? There are many important questions to look at. Write down your questions and then try to answer them on paper. Have your partner do the same exercise, but separately from you.

You will want to think of the emotional impact on your relationships with your partner, family, and friends. Will secrecy or discomfort about your pain and grief become difficult to deal with in the future? Can you build good communication and openly have differences in these relationships?

Look at both short-term and long-term needs and feelings. While it may be tempting to make a decision based on your current feelings and needs, give thought to the future. Ask yourself questions like: What will we tell our children and subsequent children? Might we have regrets that could be hard to live with? Will we be able to afford the care our child needs? What impact might this child's needs have on our family and our other children? How might we feel on birthdays and holidays? How will I reconcile my decision, given my faith? Be aware that things that seem less painful now may actually bring more pain later on. There is no guarantee. While you can never really know or prepare for this, at least give it some thought and talk about it with others who might understand.

Talk with your partner. It is likely that you will be in agreement on some aspects and have quite different feelings about others. This topic will be addressed in further detail later.

Look within yourself. What do you feel in your heart? This probably is the most important aspect of your decision. You will want to carefully consider your values, traditions, religious needs, physical needs, family needs and your baby. Once you have gathered enough background information, ask yourself how you feel about it all. Trust your feelings. Listen to your inner self. This is the vital personal and emotional component.

How certain are we about the diagnosis?

"This was my problem: I had one week to decide. The first question out of my mouth was, 'Could the test be wrong?'" Joette

If you do not feel very confident of the diagnosis or are confused, **do not make a decision to end or continue the pregnancy at this moment.** Ask your medical caregiver to give you something in writing about the test results and the problem they have found. Maybe they have an article or brochure on this problem. If there is no medical literature available, have the diagnosis written down. Anything in writing will help you remember what was said and later seek more information from other sources.

At this point you may ask for further testing, more information and/or seek a second opinion. This too is your right. Physicians and other medical practitioners usually encourage this approach. In fact, in many states two to three opinions and multiple tests are required before a decision to terminate can be made.

When talking with your care provider about the tests, you will want to know the difference between a screening and a diagnostic test. You will also want to ask about the test's accuracy. Some of these tests, such as MSAFP, are screening, not diagnostic and if the results are abnormal they need follow-up. Level I ultrasound by itself can be diagnostic, but is usually for screening purposes. Rarely does it provide enough information to make an accurate diagnosis of the problem.

Decisions about continuing or ending the pregnancy should not be made on *one test,* especially if it is a screening test. If the results do show problems, this is a red flag to consider further testing, such as an amniocentesis or Level II ultrasound. Of course, if you do not want further tests and wish to continue the pregnancy no matter what, it is your right to refuse any further tests, although in some cases they may help you better plan for the birth of your child.

"We had many ultrasounds done. Our doctor saw a black mass that he could not explain. I then went for a higher level ultrasound. We were told that our baby had an opening on her skull with a sac out of the back of her head. It is called encephalocele. He said there was no way to tell if the sac had any brain tissue in it until after she was born. And there was no surgery that could correct it. He recommended abortion. When we left his office that day I just felt like dying. After that day I never thought again about abortion. The high risk doctors I then went to gave us hope. Chelsea Brianna was born by C-section on March 3, 1992. She did have a sac on the back of her head. Through a CT scan we knew there was about a fingertip of brain tissue in it. She went through some surgeries and everything went fine. At one month we settled down to enjoy our baby. She is now one year and walking,

talking some and is truly our miracle baby. She is at high risk for developmental delay. But so far she is right on target." Faye

"I feel that my three ultrasounds by three doctors in two hospitals gave a very accurate diagnosis of Christina's physical abnormalities. This was later confirmed by the autopsy results as well." Debra

If you are uncomfortable or confused about further testing or seek more information, contact a medical library at your local hospital or at a university medical school. Make copies of articles and bring them to your care provider for interpretation. Be aware that information in the medical library can be outdated, confusing, even frightening, and difficult to interpret. Sometimes cases that make it into the medical literature are the extreme forms of that condition. Some hospitals may not allow the public to use their medical library. A public library may also be able to help you. Even if they don't have the materials you are seeking, they may have access to them from other sources. You will want to speak with a reference librarian.

Seeking another opinion may be something you want to do but feel confused about. Think about it for awhile. If a physician suddenly said your ten-year-old son needed his leg amputated, would you immediately authorize this to be done? Or would you get a second opinion and learn as much as you could before you signed the form? If your child were in a deep coma after an accident and after one test turning off the life support was recommended, would you feel you have enough information to do this? Would you need some time to sift through the information and your feelings? It may seem like you are challenging the authority of your doctor by getting more information or another opinion. Your desire to be informed and responsible should not be threatening to him/her. If so, consider seeing another doctor.

If you feel pressured by time constraints, ask for specifics about why it is necessary to do this so fast. If your state has a limit that you are approaching, maybe a neighboring state would give you a few more days or weeks. Going elsewhere may be an option that gives you the little extra time you need, if you want to go and can afford it.

I don't want any further tests. Is that my right?

This is an important question to consider before you go any further. Either you, your partner or both of you may feel strongly that no matter what you learn from more testing you will *not* end this pregnancy. You may have your personal reasons why you don't want any more tests. Whatever your situation, it is your right to say **STOP**. You can get off

1 5

what may seem like a testing roller coaster right now. You may not want more information and, in fact, may feel that more information will only add to your stress.

Be aware that sometimes learning more is helpful if you want to be prepared for what might lie ahead. The information could affect the management of your pregnancy if you decide not to abort the baby. You may also feel that additional knowledge will give you the chance to gather support and make any necessary medical arrangements for the type of birth experience you want and the care of your newborn.

"We decided to have no more tests because it only seemed to point to the worst and we needed to try and stay positive." Monica

Talk with your partner and look inside your heart. If you intend to continue the pregnancy without further tests or procedures outside the realm of normal prenatal care, inform your care provider. Although you may feel some pressure to have more tests, you are under no obligation to do so. *Do not let other people's need for information control your decisions, but be sure you are making an informed decision.*

I do want further tests. What tests do I ask for?

Before you seek other tests or even another opinion, *find a support person* to accompany you and your partner. You will need an extra pair of ears to help remember and possibly interpret the information. When in crisis it is very common not to see clearly or hear very well. Memory may be clouded and short.

You may not be considering ending the pregnancy at all, but wish to have the tests to provide as much knowledge as possible as you prepare for what is ahead. Further testing is not just for those who are leaning toward interrupting the pregnancy.

The types of tests that can be done will depend on the problem that has been diagnosed or suspected, how far along you are in the pregnancy, the information you are seeking and how that information will contribute to your decision. For example, maternal serum alpha-fetoprotein (MSAFP) screening or other maternal serum marker screening might reveal elevated or decreased values which could mean that something is wrong with the baby, or that there are multiple babies, or an inaccurate dating of the pregnancy, or as is fairly common, a "false positive" result. This screening tool, however, will be an indicator that you may want further testing. Ultrasound results may also lead you to request more testing. A genetic counselor or medical practitioner can advise you of the possible tests you may wish to consider. Again, this will depend on the suspected problem and a number of other issues. Before and during the tests write down your concerns and questions.

Some of the possible tests are: ultrasound, also known as a sonogram, either Level I or Level II (a higher resolution and more detailed ultrasound), which can examine the head, body and internal organs, as well as monitor fetal growth and development; amniocentesis, to look for possible chromosomal or other genetic problems, and in the third trimester of pregnancy, lung maturation; fetal echocardiogram to look more closely for congenital heart problems, and a number of other fetal or maternal blood tests to look for specific problems. Each situation is so different. It is impossible to recommend or describe the many tests here, especially since technology is changing rapidly and the possible problems being looked for are so many. Your medical care provider should provide you with verbal and written information on these tests, why they are suggested, what information they provide and their statistical accuracy. <u>Ask for the information in writing.</u> It is hard to remember all of what you hear. You will also want to learn about any possible associated risks to you or your baby. These factors may affect your decision about whether or not you even want the test.

Some tests, such as amniocentesis, take time before the results will be back. The wait may seem endless and difficult. You may feel confused about whether or not to tell people about the pregnancy and whether to allow yourself to get further invested. Find at least a few people with whom you can share your fears and anxieties.

You may wonder if this problem can be fixed while the baby is still *in utero*. While this is still very rare, it is a good question to ask. There seems to be limited success with surgical intervention in disorders such as diaphragmatic hernia, obstructive hydrocephalus and some kidney and bladder malformations, for example. In the years ahead, there will undoubtedly be more breakthroughs in this very specialized area of fetal therapy.

"The three weeks it took to get the results of the amnio were the longest three weeks of my life. We did a lot of talking and thinking about what we would do if the amnio showed the problem we suspected." Shelley

There are some situations that no tests can accurately diagnose. Sometimes, even after amniocentesis, fetal blood sampling and several sonograms, the severity or certainty of a problem cannot always be predicted. Some problems, such as fluid around the heart, brain or lungs, may resolve themselves during the pregnancy. There also can be misreading or confusion when ultrasound creates an image that may be difficult to interpret. In these cases, a second opinion can be particularly helpful. There are no guarantees. This is not an exact science and pregnancy and the baby's development have not been so closely studied in large enough numbers as to be able to predict *everything* with certainty.

"Rarely a day goes by that I don't think about it. Even though through tests we ruled out several abnormalities, there was a 1 in 7 chance that Alyson would be born with a genetic syndrome that could not be diagnosed until birth, even with all the sophisticated tests. We consulted specialists, had further testing and got as much information as possible. We prayed, surrounded ourselves with supportive people and followed our hearts. I could not live with the fact that I could have terminated a healthy child. Others may not have been willing to take the chance to wait and see. We made the decision we could live with then and now. Thankfully, Alyson is 15 months old, perfect, healthy and a joy." Lynn

How do I seek another opinion?

If you feel it will be helpful to get another opinion, open communication with your medical care provider is usually the first place to start. This is not about mistrust, but rather about your needing reassurance and further information. Ask your medical care provider or insurance carrier how to proceed in getting another opinion. Usually they have a referral network and will be able to give you names of people to call. Some may even make the call for you. You could also call a local hospital or seek out the nearest perinatologist (a high risk pregnancy physician), genetic counselor or pediatrician for referral information. If birth defects are suspected and you haven't already spoken with a genetic counselor, you may want to ask for a referral to a genetic counselor, who can be an especially important source for further information, as well as an advocate for you. They have advanced training in both medical genetics and counseling. Referral information for genetic counselors can come from your hospital, doctor, the Alliance of Genetic Support Groups or the National Society of Genetic Counselors listed in the **Appendix**.

Before any medical appointments, write down all of your questions, bring any written material you have, and again, remember to *bring someone with you as a support person*. It can seem overwhelming and difficult to comprehend all that is said when in shock. Ask questions over again. Repeat back the answers or what you thought you heard. This will allow your care provider an opportunity to see whether or not you understood. Do not let big words overwhelm you. Ask to have things clarified until you think you fully understand.

I feel so out of control. What can I do to gain some back?

Losing control is something most people fear. If you maintain some control, you may feel you can handle things better. Otherwise we can feel lost, unclear about where to go and what to do next. You probably feel that you have lost much control at this point in time. The disturbing news has sent you into a tailspin. The unfairness, time pressures, societal and medical pressures, confusion about your beliefs, needs and desires and maybe even some of the uncertainty about the diagnosis may be overwhelming.

Your self-confidence may waiver. You may sense the fragility of life, and this too can be frightening. At times you may look at everyone you love and fear losing them as well. It seems there is so little you can do to take control and keep everyone healthy. You may feel like a different person. You are changed; there is no doubt.

To regain some control, you may want to take a few deep breaths and plan where to begin. Use this book as a tool in your decision making. The section on **Deciding** may be helpful to remind you of, or teach you, good skills to use when faced with a dilemma that requires a decision. While there will be many things you cannot control, search for the things you *can* control—decisions that *are* within your power.

When people ask how they can help, tell them. Give them some specific ideas, such as make a meal, watch your other children, go for a walk with you or anything else you think would be helpful. Be sure you make time to take care of yourself, if only for a half-hour each day. Get rest, take walks and stay physically active, do some fun things when you can, listen to calm music and read books to escape or for reflective reading. This will help you stay in control and keep a perspective. Trust yourself. Take this a little at a time, seek the information you need, consult with appropriate support people and then, most importantly look within your heart to determine the direction you will go.

"When told the news I felt trapped and so out of control. Our varied religious backgrounds and different views on abortion made the choices difficult. I believed Monica could only do what she could live with and

19

I must support that. She acknowledged my feelings and listened to me, which helped so I didn't feel left out." Tim

Gathering information and resources

There are voluntary organizations providing up-to-date information to parents and professionals for most genetic disorders and many other problems. The Alliance of Genetic Support Groups, listed in the **Appendix,** has an 800 number to assist you in locating an appropriate group. You may also want to track down resources affiliated with the county or state or private organizations that will offer care, financial help and sometimes even information about adoption of babies who are facing physical or mental challenges. While there might be an organization that deals with your particular situation or problem, it is almost impossible to list them all here. A few key resource centers and publications are listed in the **Appendix.**

These resources should be able to provide you with information on many issues. You could also contact a hospital, medical school, your library, a genetic counselor, a hospital or university medical library and the March of Dimes. A university medical center or large hospital in your area might have a perinatal social worker who can direct you to resources. Your medical provider should have some knowledge about these resources too and may be able to help interpret information. It's likely that some of the information you find will be written for the medical community. No doubt this will be frustrating and disappointing. Be persistent in asking for both information and explanations.

If you have gathered information from the medical literature, be sure to check the date of the publication, since the information may already be outdated.

"Our baby's syndrome was not in the public library books. We obtained medical books with our doctor's help." J.

DECIDING

"I regret being forced to make a decision at all. I feel that it is so unfair to ask that such a decision be made by a mere mortal." Sheila

The diagnosis is confirmed. How do I decide?

Once you have a good base of information, it is time to work toward a decision. Sometimes receiving too much information can cause you to feel overloaded. Try to determine which information is most significant and disregard the rest for now. You might find it helpful to write each choice at the top of a piece of paper and then list what you perceive to be the pros and cons under each choice.

Along with the facts, use your intuition and feelings. Look at the varied facts and issues involved and then sort through your feelings before you do anything hasty.

"We had a number of doctors tell us that they felt it would be 'too painful' to continue the pregnancy since the baby's prognosis was so poor. In spite of their advice we decided we could not abort the baby." Bob and Suzanne

"We made a list of pros and cons for having quadruplets versus twins. We included issues such as: finances, work, family, child care, health risks and how each decision made us feel. It was the most difficult decision we have ever had to make." Jan

"When originally faced with the decision to continue or terminate my pregnancy, I concentrated mostly on three things: 1) how I felt I could deal with a baby with severe physical defects, 2) how much the attention required by this baby would take away from my two-year-old son and our marriage, and 3) what life could possibly be like for a baby with these defects. Knowing how life can be so very difficult when you are 'normal,' I knew our baby would be at a severe disadvantage. The hardest part was not knowing the extent of the disabilities; we had to make the decision based on the knowledge that our baby's arms were not developed below the elbows. A baby without hands would not be able to pull itself up, feed itself, or suck its thumb for comfort. Talking to our pediatrician helped. He talked about the other problems he has seen along with limb abnormalities." Gwen

21

Once you make your decision, you will want to feel that you are doing the right thing and that you made the best decision you could. Ask people to support you in your decision, not question or undermine it. Tell your doctor, geneticist, counselor, pastoral advisor and family that you need their support and strength to help you do what you feel you must.

"After I decided to continue the pregnancy, the geneticist kept reminding me about the statistics and possibilities of problems. I know she felt she needed to do her job, but I became so angry, feeling that she didn't respect my decision, that she was trying to take my hope away. Even though I was completely committed to my baby, her reminders increased my anxiety. I distanced myself from her to keep my sanity. I didn't need reminders about my baby's possible problems. I lived with the fears day and night. I needed hope and support to get through the pregnancy. My goal was to stay sane and to nurture my baby." Lynn

"My doctors, minister and family, the ones who knew, were fairly supportive of our decision to end the pregnancy. They knew it was for the best and the baby would not have to suffer through a lifetime of trouble and pain." J.

You might make your decision, feel relief that it is finally made, then a day or two later begin to second-guess and feel confused. You may even want to change your decision. This is natural. People do this all the time with other decisions and this type of heavy decision, too. Try not to second-guess yourself.

How to make decisions—Decision-making models

Even if you are normally good at making decisions during a crisis those skills might not readily be available to you. When faced with stressful decisions where the outcome is uncertain, it is natural to attempt to avoid making the decision, hoping the problem will go away by itself. You need to have confidence in yourself to go forward, believing that you can make the best decision possible for you at this time. To aid you in this process, this section will address making good decisions.

Suggestions for aiding you in making a decision follow. Feel free to use, change, disregard these ideas or try another method. The first model has been adapted, with a number of changes, from the book *Choices* by Shad Helmstetter (1988). Try this exercise only after you have collected as much information as you can find and can absorb. It is most helpful if you and your partner do this seperately, then compare notes.

Steps in deciding and making a choice

1. Say to yourself, "This choice is mine."
2. Write down and say out loud, "My options are_____."
3. For each choice list the positives and negatives as you see them, not as you think others will see them.
4. If there are more than two options, eliminate the ones you are not able to consider or are not interested in pursuing.
5. When you are down to two choices answer the following for each option: "I choose to_____. I decide this because_____."
6. Does one of those choices feel better in your heart?

Now talk with your partner and compare answers and feelings.

David D. Wheeler, in his book *A Practical Guide for Making Decisions* (1980), presents some basic steps in making a good decision. A few of them are:

1. Accept the challenge. You are here, you must decide and you *can* meet the challenge.
2. Search for alternatives and information.
3. Evaluate each alternative carefully, factually, spiritually and emotionally.
4. Forecast the future. Try to imagine and predict the possible implications and outcome in six months, a year and five years. Do the best you can. Of course you know that the future cannot be adequately pedicted, only guessed at.
5. Make your choice and become committed.
6. Overcome setbacks. It will not go smoothly, challenges will arise. Prepare yourself to deal with these setbacks.

A Decision-Making Exercise

A list of questions follow that could be used as a worksheet to help you stay focused on issues and your concerns/needs while at the same time listening to your partner's needs. This was adapted from work done by Sheila Maland, a mother who lived through the same dilemma you are grappling with and who now runs a support group for families who have faced this challenge.

Some ground rules to keep in mind:

- Address each question that seems pertinent to you.
- Answer in writing, not by talking. This gives each of you a chance to formulate your own opinion.
- Because this is a long exercise you may want to consider doing a few questions at a time.
- When your answers are complete, exchange papers with your partner. Take it question by question and try to verbally explain your understanding of what your partner is trying to say. If the writer has anything to add at this time, they may do so.

While this seems like a very basic and almost elementary exercise, it has a good chance of helping each of you learn the other's perspective without being interrupted, challenged, tuned-out or misinterpreted. After each person is clearly heard and feels understood, an open discussion may begin. Here are the main questions. Feel free to add others or change these, but do so by writing them down.

1. What was my view on pregnancy termination before I got the news about my child? What are my views now?

2. What are my religious, personal and family values, and how might they influence my decision? What if my decision contradicts my values?

3. What is my understanding of what my life will be like if I end this pregnancy now?

4. What is my understanding of what my life will be like if I continue the pregnancy and the baby dies on its own prior to, during or shortly after birth?

5. If this child lives beyond birth, how might my life be changed physically, emotionally, spiritually and financially? How might my relationship with my mate and my other children be affected?

6. What type of life do I envision this child having? During the first year, ages 1-5, 5-10, 10-20, 20+? Are my impressions based on things I have observed, read or heard from others? Do I feel comfortable with this information?

7. How might this decision affect my life during the time frames listed above? Where did I get this information? What have I observed, read or felt? Where can I get more information?

8. What is my worst fear? Is it that the child will die or that s/he will live and be severely challenged? If my worst fear comes true, what will I need from myself, my partner and others to make it through this?

9. How do I envision communicating my decision either to continue or to end the pregnancy—to family, friends and co-workers?

10. Who do I think would be there as a support network for me if I end the pregnancy? If I carry the pregnancy to term? If the baby lives past birth?

11. If my decision is to interrupt the pregnancy, what method of termination do I think would be best? Why? What things would I like to make sure are done at the time of the loss (e.g. seeing the baby, holding a funeral service?) More information on this important aspect can be found in the section **Hello, Goodbye**.

12. If I decide to continue the pregnancy what are my options and what will help me during the rest of the pregnancy, at the birth and in the future if the baby lives?

13. For some couples, this pregnancy may have been the culmination of years of infertility treatment or previous losses, or it may be the last chance for pregnancy because of age or for other reasons. Is carrying a pregnancy to term an important goal? If so, why?

14. Putting all rational thoughts aside, in my heart what do I think is the best decision—for my unborn child, for me, for my family?

After you and your partner have answered these questions, compare your answers and seek to understand or at least listen to each other, even if you don't agree.

What if my partner and I disagree?

You and your partner may find it hard to agree on exactly what to do, when to do it, or even how to proceed at this moment. One of you may question the idea of termination, while the other is convinced that there is no other option. One of you may want to tell relatives and friends while the other may not. Unfortunately, there is no compromise or middle ground to this very serious decision. *Not to decide is to decide.* Even if you normally communicate quite well, you may find yourself frustrated when talking with your partner about this important issue. Perhaps you are having difficulty concentrating and really listening to each other. When one has struggled with an intense decision it might be especially difficult to acknowledge other points of view.

This situation can put a serious strain on your relationship. Maybe you don't feel you can explain your thoughts well or don't wish to share some personal views that are hard for you to state. This can be frustrating and overwhelming. You may feel inadequately prepared to deal with such a life and death decision, especially if the answer is not at all clear or there is strong disagreement. Be careful not to add to your hurt by saying things to each other you don't mean. Or you might find yourselves agreeing on more things than you would have expected, yet it is still stressful. Consider seeking help from an outside support person such as a spiritual advisor, a genetic counselor or a therapist to help keep you focused on the issue at hand and work with you in problem solving.

You might wish to read more on the differences in grieving between men and women in the section entitled **Do men and women grieve differently?**

"I feared Bob and I were going to disagree. In my uncertainty I almost didn't want to verbalize some of my thoughts." Suzanne

"I was conscious of the fact that she would have the physical burden of our decision. I restrained from making any strong statements so as not to influence Suzanne. I could not force her, it really had to be a decision she would be comfortable with, yet it wasn't just her decision. But I worried, what if we disagreed? What if she decided to abort? Could I live with that?" Bob

"I was strongly leaning toward ending the pregnancy, but I realized that in the end it really had to be Monica's decision, since she was carrying the baby and would be the one to feel its life end. We went with her choice. I was okay with that." Tim

I am single and don't have an involved partner to help me.

In this difficult time you might need support from someone. Making this decision all by yourself can be very difficult, though certainly not impossible. If that is what you have to do or choose to do, you *can* do it! However, if you want support, think about the people you trust—a parent, relative, good friend, clergyperson and/or co-worker. Is there someone who supports you, listens to you and does not challenge or undermine your decisions? That is the type of person you need. Seek them out and tell him or her what is happening. If you feel good about their response, ask them to be with you during meetings with your medical team and invite them to be your sounding board as you work toward a decision.

I feel pressure from others to make a certain decision.

Whether it is subtle or direct, you will find that some people express their own strong beliefs about what they think you should or should not do. They probably realize that you are agonizing over your decision and they want to help you move on. It may seem easy for someone to think they know what to do or what they think is best for you, but only *you* can make your decision. Someone might suggest, for example, that a death would be less painful than the daily demands of raising a seriously disabled child. They may indeed feel that death would be easier to deal with, but they don't know what *you* think and they can never walk in your shoes. Until your decision is made, some people might feel it is their responsibility to give you advice and influence. If you don't want this, communicate your desire to be spared from their advice.

No one can magically make you feel better or make the best decision for you now. However, please know that others care about you and want what is best for you. They want you to have the least amount of pain necessary, to "get over this" quickly and they hope you will make a speedy recovery. It is often this caring that leads others to try to guide or direct you in your decision making. If there are a few people who appear to be cruel or who misunderstand, don't let them affect you negatively. They have the attitude problem, not you. Trust yourself and *be gentle with yourself* during this confusing time.

"Most said to abort now, don't prolong the personal agony. I was told by a woman to 'get rid of it!'" M.

"Prior to this experience my husband and I were firm in our beliefs about abortion and the sanctity of life. The doctors were very strong and persuasive in their reasoning. They encouraged us to terminate our pregnancy, advising it would be too painful emotionally for me to carry the baby full-term. I found myself wavering. Bob wavered less than I, and in a short time we did decide to continue the pregnancy." Suzanne

How do I use my conscience, faith, ethics and values to make this decision?

"The first and most important step for us was talking with our pastor. He addressed three aspects of the decision that we would need to deal with—spiritual, psychological and physical. While I was very much afraid of the physical pain I knew it would be temporary and bearable. I felt in a lot of ways I had dealt with the psychological issues, so the pastor's presence got us through the spiritual aspect." Gwen

Your upbringing and moral code will influence your decision and your response afterwards. The intensity of your beliefs will likely relate to the intensity of your reactions. You might be opposed to abortion, yet you find yourself considering abortion. Or you might have been accepting of abortion for others but now wonder if it is acceptable for you. The reality of your situation is very different than you ever could have anticipated. This new situation might challenge you spiritually and morally. You are on a very personal journey; one that can never be easy. Seek the support you need, looking deeply at who *you* are and what you feel is best or necessary to do. Be kind to yourself and your partner. Take time off from work if possible. Find solace, listen to music, go for walks, talk or write about this, pray and let out your tears and fears. Find the best way to express yourself as you explore your faith and values. Trust in your ability to decide what is the better option for you and your family.

"I was so against abortion that I believed it would never even be a consideration. Now, via ultrasound, I was faced with a baby whose life could not continue once the cord was cut. I have learned to never say 'never' for life changes us in many ways." J.

"In our hearts we knew that we couldn't abort a child even if the problem was very serious. During the difficult decision-making times I prayed continuously for guidance. While my husband wavered occasionally, I remained in favor of continuing the pregnancy. Since it was my body and I was so insistent, Jim supported me in my choice." M.

Trust in your faith, God and your intuition. Believe that you have the strength and faith to survive. A positive and trusting attitude will go a long way now. While you are trying to gain control, also work on letting go of control. Maybe much of this really is out of your hands. It might not seem easy, but you *are coping*, and with calmness and trust you will go forward to brighter days.

THE OPTIONS

As you explore your options carefully, you might find the following information helpful. The next two main sections are **Continuing the Pregnancy** and **Terminating the Pregnancy**. **Selective reduction** is found within the section **Terminating the Pregnancy**. Feel free to read only what you want to read, just skip the pages that aren't for you. If you want a sense of the bigger picture and wish to consider all of your options, read all or just parts of each section. Even if your exact situation is not described, feel included and read what fits.

"My baby had a kidney disease; he would die a few hours after birth. Since I was eight months pregnant I did not have the option of termination. I was devastated that I would have to carry the baby to term. I wondered how I would survive carrying around a baby who was going to die. Davon William was born at 36 weeks. To this day I am very grateful I did not have to make that decision on whether to end the pregnancy. I got to hold my son, kiss him and love him, and so did many of my family members. My son brought me more love from so many people that I otherwise never would have felt so deeply. I also liked the fact that I could tell him when he was inside me that I loved him no matter what, that he was my baby." Mary

"When they told us there was something wrong with one of the twins that might endanger the other's life we were in shock. How could this be? We struggled with our decision, knowing that we really had no choice. Ending that baby's life was the hardest thing we ever did." Terry

"Our perfect baby was perfect no more. After one standard ultrasound our bubble was burst. Could we, would we end our baby's life, our very loved and wanted baby? How cruel that we were even in a position where we had to contemplate this!" Chris

"For two years we went through test after test, trying to have a baby. After artificial insemination we learned at six week's gestation that we were to have FIVE babies! It was inconceivable, in my wildest dreams I never thought I would have more than one baby. Amidst the excitement we had a serious problem. Having five babies was next to impossible, so we had to make a decision. How many babies should we have? This was not a choice I should have been making. Who was I to play God and choose which babies would die or live?" Susan

CONTINUING THE PREGNANCY

Why do people continue the pregnancy?

They continue because:
- "I hoped the tests were wrong."
- "I needed to feel I did everything to give my baby the best chance. We love her dearly and will help her live for as long as she can."
- "There was no choice. The time had passed for a legal abortion. My baby had Potter syndrome and I was 28 weeks when I found out."
- "We didn't want to play God. Who were we to decide what should happen to our baby's life? We had to trust that what was meant to be would happen."
- "We don't believe in abortion, for any reason. We didn't think we could live with ourselves if we ended the pregnancy."
- "I decided I could accept a less than perfect baby. After awhile the diagnosis didn't sound so bad to me. At least the baby would probably live. We can deal with this. We have a lot of love to give."
- "I wasn't convinced that the diagnosis was accurate. Though my husband and I disagreed about this, it turned out our baby was really okay. I am so thankful."
- "One of our twins was gravely ill at 18 week's gestation. We could not terminate her life even though her twin might not have been harmed by the procedure."
- "We learned that there were loving families who would care for a handicapped child. This gave us the courage to go ahead with the pregnancy, keeping that option as an *out* if it became too hard for us to take care of our baby."
- "The diagnosis wasn't absolute. It was a syndrome that could not be identified 100 percent until after birth. The amnio and ultrasounds encouraged us since the vital organs were well developed. We could not terminate a baby that might have been healthy. We decided to take our chances."
- "Even though our baby died shortly after birth, I am glad we let the pregnancy go to term. At least we had a whole baby to touch, see, dress and take pictures of. We have those very special memories of the pregnancy and our baby. They are comforting to us now."
- "My baby could possibly have been a miracle baby! Of course the doctors were saying that there was no way the baby would survive, but I felt that possibly a miracle could happen. This could be our miracle baby!"
- "I was afraid of all the technology. I rebelled against it and waited too long to make the decision. That allowed me to have a few months

where I could act like it was a somewhat normal pregnancy. As hard as it was at times, I have no regrets."

Is adoption an alternative if I feel I cannot raise this child?

There might be adoption agencies and group homes in your area or state that can provide loving homes for children who are physically impaired or mentally challenged, even severely so. This can be an alternative that allows you to continue the pregnancy and keep your options open, until you see how the baby is. You could make some contacts ahead of time so you are prepared, but hold off signing anything unless you are absolutely sure of the baby's condition and your inability to parent this child. Once your baby is born, you can speak with your partner and your doctor and use your support system to determine if you want to try parenting or wish to give your baby up to another family for adoption. There are often waiting lists of people who are willing to love and care for children who have problems. The **Appendix** lists a national adoption organization that can link you with state and local resources.

"I recently terminated my pregnancy because my baby had Down syndrome. The doctor told me I could either continue the pregnancy or end it. He then went into all the details of the abortion. We decided to interrupt the pregnancy. Then later we learned that in our state there was a waiting list of families wanting to adopt a baby with Down's. If I had known this I might have made a different decision. While I am not sure about this, I think I should at least have been told the whole story. This would have been more fair and unbiased. Instead I feel I was pressured to look at termination. We did not think we wanted to raise a Down's baby." A.

Can the doctors be wrong? Might the baby survive and live a fairly normal life?

In a limited number of situations, a diagnosis that looked certain or fairly certain during pregnancy turned out to be wrong when the baby was born. Perhaps the ultrasound showed serious problems early on, but those problems went away later in pregnancy. Or maybe the condition diagnosed was actually found to be less severe than expected after birth. Many people have felt so strongly about prayer and positive thought that they believed, through these thoughts or their faith in God, their baby could be healed. Some parents have had a very strong feeling that their baby was fine, no matter what the tests indicated. Maybe the mother had a problem that led some medical professionals to suggest termination or selective reduction to save the life of some of the babies, yet all the babies lived. This is not a perfect science, things can change in the pregnancy. Though this is not commonplace, it does happen. You will decide whether or not to take that chance.

"No one could tell me how selective reduction would affect the surviving babies. Was there more of a chance of miscarriage if I had the procedure? No one could answer the questions. They believed there probably would not be an increased risk, but there were no guarantees." Susan

When you get other opinions, investigate the information and seek support. It's okay to rely on your faith if that is what is right for you. It may work out or it may not. Unfortunately, no one can look into the future and accurately predict how your circumstances will turn out. If you decide on non-intervention, for whatever reason, do get the medical and emotional support you need to continue on the course you choose. You have traveled down unknown roads before and have made it, and you can adapt to what is ahead on this journey also.

"In our second pregnancy we were told that I had toxoplasmosis. Abortion was proposed by several people. My own doctor researched it and repeatedly assured and advised me that we could treat it with medication and the baby would be normal. We got a second opinion and relied on our physician and our personal strength and determination. Our son is normal, healthy and wonderful. In this case, the assurances that the problem could be overcome (with still a risk, of course) were so positive that we decided not to abort." M.

"Even though several specialists said it didn't look good, I knew in my heart I didn't want to abort my baby, who we learned would be a girl, our Maggie. Her lungs might not support her after birth, but I wanted to give her that chance. Maybe they were wrong, maybe it would get better, if we prayed hard, and if she were strong enough. Though she wasn't supposed to live, Maggie Louise Mullenmaster is now a very strong one-year-old. Thank God I listened to my inner heart. They might have been right and Maggie might have died, but at least I would have a full nine months of her alive inside me that no one could take away." Monica

There are a growing number of support groups, literature sources and organizations for people who are parenting a child with problems, even though it sometimes seems we don't value these children as a society. Seek support and referrals if you don't think you can do the day-to-day parenting. There may be financial support available also, if this is a concern. The listings in the **Appendix**, your county social service offices and your hospital social worker are a few places you could check to learn about resources in your area.

"When we were 21 weeks pregnant, a sonogram showed multiple abnormalities of the heart, spine and kidneys. The physician expected the baby to die within three weeks. After the first shock wore off I thought about abortion. My husband did not. I did not want to endure the pain of waiting; I desperately wanted an easy way out. I'm glad I took my time in deciding what to do. Within a week I had decided to let the pregnancy continue. Morally, I simply could not end my child's life. What about my conscience? Although my child's life would be ended, mine would not. How could I ever escape the guilt of not giving my child an opportunity to live? J.

"By the following week we had decided we would see our child no matter how disabled he was. By the next week we knew that his big brother would have to see him as well. Each week gave us more time to plan. Frank was born at 38 weeks. It was a long and painful wait; but he gave us this great gift of life, even if it was only for a few minutes. He gave us his love and in turn we gave ours. He was a beautiful son. He taught us about unconditional love, patience, endurance and strength. We were fortunate in that we were able to say hello before we said goodbye." Cubby

What if I change my mind and just can't wait for the baby to be born naturally?

Before you make the decision to continue the pregnancy you might want to ask, "What if I can't take it any longer and want to change my mind?" In most states there are laws that will allow the physician to induce labor only up to a certain number of weeks. Under some circumstances exceptions can be made to the rules. Unless your baby has died or your own health is in serious jeopardy, you probably will not be able to change your mind and end the pregnancy once you are past the number of weeks allowed by your state or other states to which you might travel for the termination to be done. Be aware of all of these options.

There is no way to tell how long your pregnancy and the birth process will last. It can depend on what is wrong with the baby, the gestational age of the baby, if there are multiples, or how the mother is doing. In some cases, the baby is born naturally soon after the problem is diagnosed; in others it may take weeks or even months. For instance, it is believed that without induction, anencephalic babies are often born after their due dates, since the brain-secreted hormones necessary to induce labor are absent. Prolonging pregnancy occasionally can become a health hazard to the mother. As with any pregnancy you might go past your due date. There are no time guarantees. Your medical care providers will want to monitor your pregnancy as it nears term, making sure you don't develop any complications. They will be able to tell you if they think things are changing in your body, and might then discuss what the options are at that point.

If your baby has died your doctor might want to induce labor. The description of the procedures likely to be used can be explained by your doctor or genetic counselor. They are also briefly described in the section called **Terminating the Pregnancy**. You will want to find supportive people to assist you throughout the induction and delivery, as well as in the days to follow. The section **Hello, Goodbye** offers ideas for creating special memories and learning about your options during this difficult time. A support group or organization that assists families to cope with infant death can also be helpful. See the **Appendix** for a list.

How do I tell people?

If you choose to continue the pregnancy there may be many who breathe a sigh of relief and do their best to support you. No doubt there will be those who tell you that they could never cope with something like this. You might be praised for being brave while you are feeling just the opposite. Some are bound to ask why you don't just end the pregnancy and be done with it. You may feel angry at these people. Their sense of pain and fear for you, and their own imaginings of how difficult it would be for them to cope under these circumstances are influencing their judgment of you. It might seem as if they are questioning your decision. Do not allow them to undermine your confidence. What they don't understand is that any choice available to you brings pain and heartache. Share your decision with them and emphasize that it is final. That way they should feel less free to try to influence you.

Remind yourself that you are making the best decision for you and your family at this time. *You* will have to live with yourself and the consequences, *they won't..* Try to surround yourself with the people who support your decision. Avoid people who are unsupportive or cause you to be uncomfortable, even if they are family members. This is a time to put your blinders on. Allow people to have their opinions, but do not allow them to affect yours.

"My family was not able to be supportive of our decision to continue the pregnancy. They said things like, 'How can you put us through this. Why don't you just end it now?'" Cindy

Many questions might arise. Should you avoid people so you don't have to explain about the baby every time they see your growing belly? Do you go about your business acting as if nothing has changed? What do you say to unsuspecting people who ask about the baby, in the grocery or movie line, at church or in a public place? You may want to scream or shout about how unfair all of this is, but another part of you may want to hide the painful truth. How you respond will depend on your mood, who is around, how much time you have, who asked and your investment in your relationship with that person.

There are no perfect or absolute answers to these uncomfortable questions. Everyone handles this differently. Most people admit that they aren't sure how they managed to survive, but they did. Trust your heart! Do what you must even if others don't fully understand and are uncomfortable. You aren't obligated to give full explanations when you don't feel like it. At other times, confiding in others will give them an opportunity to empathize with you.

"When I was asked when my baby was due, I would say something like 'In June' on the days I didn't feel like talking about it. On other days, when I wanted them to know what I was going through, I'd say, 'In June our baby may be born with severe problems. This is not an easy time for us.'" M.

"I had the greatest conversation with a store owner when she asked 'When is your baby due?' I told her the truth, with tears in my eyes and she asked all about it, offered her sincere condolences and shared her heart. I was really moved and felt better having shared my pain that day." S.

At some point, you may want to alert other people to what is happening. You can ask a friend or relative to share the news with certain people. This is emotionally draining and your energy levels may already be low. You might want to let many people or only a few know what is happening. Be honest and open about your needs whether they include books and resources, meals, childcare help, taking walks or whatever else might help. Making multiple copies of a personal card or note will allow you to tell many people at once, rather than trying to personally connect with every single person. An example of how to share your news follows:

"We are deeply saddened to share some important news about our pregnancy. Our beloved baby has severe problems and...*(you could use phrases such as the following)* • may die before or at birth • is expected to have major problems that could be life threatening • we fear for her/his health. We ask for your understanding and sensitivity during the rest of our pregnancy. This won't be an easy time for us and we will need your support. We would appreciate it if you could.... • stop by to talk with us • keep us in your prayers • still share in our pregnancy as we try to celebrate and enjoy the rest of this precious little life. Please ask us about our baby, since we will want to talk about him/her. But do understand that there will be days or moments when we won't be able to talk. We appreciate your prayers/thoughts during this difficult time."

The pregnancy and birth—how to cope

Perhaps you have no choice in this matter because you are past the deadline for legal termination and you must carry the pregnancy to its natural outcome. Or maybe after careful consideration you chose to continue the pregnancy. Regardless of the path which led you to your current circumstance, it is essential that you continue to use your support network to meet your emotional needs and keep gathering the information and resources necessary to prepare you and your family for your baby and what is to come.

Waiting through the duration of your pregnancy will be difficult. During the pregnancy, your baby is still alive, though s/he may be born with multiple problems. Many people admit feeling thankful for this extra amount of time with their baby before birth. The baby is still under their care, in its mother's womb. This waiting time may actually be helpful in beginning to work through some of the grief. Many mothers have commented that they were not ready to "let go" of their baby yet. They needed more time to protect, provide a safe and warm haven, and love, smile and cry over their baby.

You may wish to escape day-to-day routines because they suddenly seem impossible to handle. Perhaps taking a leave from your job and "hibernating" for awhile sounds good. You may want to stay home and face the challenges, while making plans for the upcoming birth. Give yourself time for privacy and for grieving. Or you may feel that the routine of work keeps you "sane" and enables you to push back reality for hours each day, so work is the best place for you. The evenings and nights may be the hardest time. Writing in a journal, listening to soothing music, and doing projects that keep you busy can offer outlets and/or distractions at this time. Sharing your love, songs and prayers with the baby can be special and can help in making precious memories for the future.

During this stressful time even small tasks can seem unmanageable. To keep yourself from becoming too overwhelmed, consider asking someone to stay with you for awhile during the pregnancy and/or after the birth to help out. You may not want to receive too many visitors or personally answer every call from people offering help. Maybe you could find someone to screen the offers of help and make suggestions to callers as to what they can do to assist you.

Finding support right now is of utmost importance. You will want to find people who will grieve with you, who will be open about what you are going through and what is to come. Much is out of your control, making your situation even more difficult to endure.

"During those 17 weeks that we waited for our baby to be born our emotions were up and down. At times we 'hid.' Other times it was therapeutic to tell people our baby would die. It helped us face the reality of it all." Cubby

"We talked with friends, made plans for a baby who would live and for one who would die, just in case either happened. I prayed a lot, asked my family and friends to pray for our baby, and kept fairly busy. When I needed my private time I could find it, since I was at home during this time. I sang and talked to the baby, made gifts and tried to embrace my pregnancy and baby to the best of my ability at the time. Thus, I have no regrets about how I handled this difficult, yet precious time." M.

A time of waiting can become a constructive time for planning when you are ready for that. As the initial shock subsides you may find this time valuable in planning and preparing for your baby's birth, and special needs or any other desires you may have. You may want to think about getting an ultrasound picture as a keepsake and even taking more pictures at the time of your delivery. See the **Hello, Goodbye** section. Consideration can also be given to preparations for a special funeral service if death occurs. You may want to buy or do something special for yourself and/or the baby. This will be a memory to cherish in days to come, no matter what happens. Though it may seem hard to believe, you *will* be able to face these difficult decisions and realities.

Depending on the type of problem and the circumstances, it is possible that your baby might die at some point during the pregnancy. You may never be ready for this, even if you were aware that this could happen. If you want to prepare yourself further, you can contact organizations or groups that deal with this, as well as seek out reading materials. This is your beloved baby and you will want to remember her or him in as many special ways as possible.

One mother called an infant loss support program and stated,*"Calling you today is the hardest thing I have ever done. I am admitting to myself, and now to you, that the baby I am carrying will most likely die. I need to know how to plan a beautiful funeral tribute. This has been my worst fear that the baby will die. And only today, after two weeks, am I ready to begin to face it. My husband's worst fear, however, has been that the baby will live and be severely handicapped. To him, death would be the lesser of two evils. Will you please tell me about the resources and give me advice on preparing for my baby's death? Also, for my husband, can you point us in the direction of resources in case our child lives but has problems?"* N.

Living through the pregnancy can seem like a long process. Your fears and concerns have the potential to be overwhelming. Try to keep calm by staying busy, trying to enjoy the pregnancy and living each day to the fullest. Take time for yourself and each other. Try to be optimistic when you can. Find a few supportive people to be there for you. Make every effort to have normal days where you don't think about your fears. If you believe in prayer or meditation, use them to gain calm and hope.

You may want to discuss a birth plan with your medical care provider. The birth may be something you worry about. Given the circumstances, what will help this be the best birth that it can be? Will your baby live? Will you get time with your baby? Who will support you? While in the hospital have someone with you for moral support. Trust and believe that you will make it, the time with your baby will be special and you will be able to go on from here.

Be sure to read the section **Hello, Goodbye** for ideas on how to experience your little one, if sh/e does die. You may want to ask if organ donation is a possibility if the idea interests you. This can be one small way to make something positive of this tragedy. Only a few infant organs, usually just the eyes, can even be considered for donation.

"At Maggie's birth I realized I had protected myself for so long that I was in shock when everything was okay. I couldn't really be excited because I had prepared for four months to be devastated." Tim

One mother was very upset that her doctor and friends appeared to think she was strange because she had decided to continue the pregnancy, though her baby would probably die shortly after birth. In addition, she asked her doctor for a Caesarean section so that her fragile baby would not be harmed during the birth and she could hold him while still alive. The doctor did not understand her reasoning, which may not have appeared rational to him, but which was in fact a loving, motherly response.

What are my rights and options if my baby lives and needs medical care?

Your rights as a parent are an important area of concern to consider when it comes to medical intervention *after* your baby is born. At what point do you no longer have a say about your child's care? What if you need to say at some point, "Don't use heroic efforts with our baby?" "Enough is enough." "Turn off the machines." Will your medical team support your wishes? Will they insist on going to all lengths to save or be legally bound to this child? Will you have to stand by helplessly without power to stop such heroic efforts? What are the financial costs? What does your insurance/health plan cover: a normal delivery, a termination, the Neonatal Intensive Care Unit or extra care your baby may need? Discuss your rights with a neonatologist, social worker or pediatrician. Most hospitals have an ethics committee which can be convened for parents to voice their wishes and learn more about their rights, options and hospital policies.

You may want to ask questions about your financial obligations and the possibilities that may lie ahead. Also be sure to discuss your coverage with your medical provider/insurance company *before* you decide, so you will better know your financial risks.

Parenting a challenged child

Depending on the baby's problems, it might not be easy parenting a child with emotional or physical difficulties. You may fear that it will be too hard, draining and unfair to the rest of the family. It is possible that this will be one of the more difficult things you have had to face. The added stress will be something for you and your family to discuss and find ways to deal with. How stable are things now? Do you feel that you will be able to pull together in the days ahead as you make a commitment to your new baby?

While frustration, sadness and sorrow are elements of parenthood, especially when parenting children with challenges, many parents discuss the joys and beauty their child has brought to the whole family. This is the side of living with disabilities that is often misunderstood and not openly discussed. Parenthood itself brings mixed blessings. Parenting a child who has problems is not always easy and happy, but it is not always sad and overwhelming either. Find the support you need. Check with your local March of Dimes chapter, a physician, The Alliance of Genetic Support Groups or the First Call For Help organization to find support groups and/or other families who have parented children with similar problems. You are not alone and need not do this by yourself. One of the first things you will want to learn is to ask for help from your relatives, friends and your community. Many may feel blessed by the positives and joy that can come from sharing in the care of a special child.

"When we learned our child would be a Down's child, it was our worst fear. The fear of the unknown is the worst. I kept thinking that I would be stuck in the house and we worried about the medical costs...you're horrified. You only concentrate on the negative. You don't realize there's going to be any quality of life at all...but it's not one percent as bad as I thought it would be. I thought she probably wouldn't have any friends. She would never celebrate birthdays. We would never laugh; we would never have a good time. But when we celebrated her second birthday in June, we had forty-five people fill the house...Katie has been a real blessing." Karen and Jim (Granat 1991)

"Parenting Andrew has been exceedingly hard at times. He needs so much care and this takes time. Sometimes I feel trapped." Nancy

What if my child dies? How will I go on living?

You may wonder how you will go on living if your child has died. No matter how it has happened, you will be left feeling empty and alone. There may be days when you feel you are going crazy. People might not understand your pain and sorrow. They may underestimate the attachment you had for this baby. Concentration may be difficult and you may feel overwhelmed. You or family members may be angry at God, each other, the medical team or at yourselves. Anger is a natural way of expressing the hurt and sadness. When you love someone and they die, the grief that follows can be very intense and uncontrollable at times.

As hard as it may seem, allow the grief to fill you and wash over you now. You loved your baby and s/he is worth grieving for and remembering. This little treasure has changed you and you will never be the same, the person you were before. While this may seem sad and hard to accept, seek a new normal, since you are now a different person. Your child has not brought you only pain and sorrow. Spend some time thinking of the good memories, the happiness, the hopes and the dreams.

You need never stop loving your baby. Cry as hard and long as you need to, express your anger, disappointment, sorrow and sadness in whatever ways you must. These feelings need to come out. That is how you will heal. Find some way to move the pain from the inside to the outside of your body, through music, prayer, physical activities, sculpting, writing, building, painting or drawing. Feel it and express it when appropriate, then put it away when you need a break. Trust yourself and be yourself.

If you ever feel seriously suicidal or have a plan for ending your life, immediately seek help from a crisis hotline, your physician or a counselor.

There are a number of books that can support you during this time, as well as many support groups. The **Appendix** has an extensive list. *Empty Arms* (Ilse 1982/1990), *When Hello Means Goodbye* (Schiebert 1979) and *Empty Cradle, Broken Heart* (Davis 1991) are good books to guide you during this difficult time.

TERMINATING THE PREGNANCY

Why do caring people choose to end a pregnancy?

They choose to terminate a pregnancy because:
- "We made the decision out of love for our baby."
- "We didn't want the baby to suffer, either physically or emotionally throughout her life."
- "Included in our decision was consideration of all of the other lives this baby would affect, such as my husband's, children's and mine. The decision to end his life was what we thought was the best one, the most caring and responsible decision we could make, the one that seemed to create the most good and prevent the most suffering."
- "I was afraid my other children would suffer because this baby would require so much extra attention and care."
- "We felt it was best for our family and the baby to end the pregnancy as soon as possible."
- "We felt we wouldn't be able to cope with the stress of having a child in intensive care for at least 6 months! We didn't want our child to suffer through multiple surgeries."
- "I knew that if my child was born alive, everything medically possible would have to be done to keep her alive. I feared that I would no longer have any say about her quality of life. I just couldn't put her through that agony when it was so hopeless."
- "I chose to terminate the pregnancy because the chance of it going to term was slim to none and because I could not continue to carry the baby knowing that he would miscarry naturally."
- "When we learned we were expecting five babies we wanted desperately to give at least some of our children a chance to live. It was so painful and unnatural choosing which babies would live and which would die."
- "I did not want to terminate the pregnancy. Not me! I believe in the value of life. But I had no amniotic fluid and the doctors said the baby had no chance of surviving. I was so confused, but I finally agreed."
- "I wanted to get this over with as soon as I could. I couldn't stand being pregnant knowing the baby might die or would be severely handicapped."
- "I was afraid of becoming even more attached to this new life and then when the birth came, I would be even more mentally messed up than I already was."
- "We did it because we loved him enough to let him go. Because of our ages, 40 and 42, we wouldn't live forever to care for him."

42

- "Neither of us believes in abortion. We didn't think ending a pregnancy would be something we would ever do or even have to consider. Yet, when faced with it and the other bad alternatives, we realized we had to choose termination."
- "A friend told us about the chronic challenges of raising a mentally retarded child. We felt we couldn't handle that. Instead we are dealing with grief after her death, but maybe there will be an end to that."
- "I knew that my baby would die at birth. I knew I was the only thing keeping my baby alive. I agonized over what to do. I was her life support system. Then I thought of my living children and the choice I would make if they were brain dead and living on a life support system. I knew I would respect them enough to recognize when their life was over."

Selective Reduction

If you are pregnant with multiple babies, usually four or more, you may need to decide whether to continue the pregnancy or selectively terminate some of the babies. Even if you had discussed this possiblility previously, it may seem shocking to consider, especially if you have been trying desperately to become pregnant in the first place. While there are no guarantees, ask about the real statistics about survival in both cases. Through this procedure some babies are randomly injected, which may result in some or all of the other children dieing. This is still a relatively new procedure that you will need to learn about. Both options have problems and no one can predict the outcome.

Chances are likely you have planned and even worked to get pregnant with these babies. The increasing use of modern reproductive technologies has made pregnancies with multiple babies more commonplace. You might have been an IVF patient, on fertility drugs or of an age where your risks for multiples was greater. Maybe at first you were elated and felt thankful that you were blessed with more than one baby. Or maybe you were surprised and dismayed. You may be confused and angry, even at your fertility specialist. Will you let nature take its course and accept the risks to the mother and the pregnancy, or does the other option sound like a better one? You will have to be the one to decide, the one to look within your heart and know what you can live with. You may want to contact larger multiple organizations (listed in the Appendix) who have supported families who have made both choices to discuss your options.

The issues you are dealing with are involve the termination or continuation issues, yet are somewhat more complicated. One of the lifelong complications will be that although you probably will feel thankful to have the children you do, your living children might be reminders of those whose lives were sacrificed. You will need support and understanding. The Pen Parents Network, listed in the **Appendix**, is a good resource to find other parents who "have been there."

"I was so thankful they took pictures during the ultrasound and gave us a copy. It is the only picture of the babies all together. This has become an important keepsake. Someday it will be helpful as I show my two sons their siblings and explain how they gave their lives that Josh and Jeremy could live." N.

"Even though the doctors strongly recommended we abort at least two of the babies, we just couldn't make that choice. We decided to let happen what was to happen. We have no regrets." B.

The idea of causing harm or hurt to my child goes against nature and my sense of what is right.

Seeing your child suffer is the ultimate heartache for you, the parent. Of course, you want the best for your baby. The thought of terminating the pregnancy and ending your baby's life might go against your every belief and value. However, as you weigh your options and the possible pain your baby may have to endure, it may seem like the lesser of two difficult choices. Some resources do exist to support you, though not very many at this point in time. There are a few groups around the country. More literature is being written, and there is a growing understanding of the intensity of the pain of this very difficult experience. Two good booklets that deal mostly with termination are: *A Time to Decide, A Time to Heal* and *Difficult Decisions*. Both are referenced in the **Bibliography**.

I don't like the word abortion.

For many people, the word abortion causes a strong emotional reaction. You may have similar feelings; it may offend you. This is under-standable. You loved this baby, you wanted him/her to live, yet you have felt it necessary to end the pregnancy.

The word abortion might be used often at this time and in days to come. It might be used interchangeably with *interrupt the pregnancy* and *terminate the pregnancy*. Even the word termination may be hard for you to hear. Medical caregivers might say abortion often; the forms you must sign and even the bill you receive once you are home are likely to list this procedure as an abortion. The medical community uses the word *abortion*, which means the early ending of a pregnancy, whether the process is natural or induced. While this might explain its use, it doesn't necessarily take into account the feelings of patients like you.

The choice of words does not change the reality of what has happened. Maybe you cannot and should not be protected from these words, though they are hard to hear. On the other hand, if it will help you, speak to your caregivers, your family and friends about your feelings and preference of what words to use. Perhaps they will be able to be sensitive to your desires. If you prefer to use another word such as "termination" or "interruption," tell them. Be prepared that the rest of the world may not accommodate you. While this has the potential to add to your pain, it might not be as traumatic if you are aware and try to prepare yourself. Just be careful not to think that by avoiding the word you can also avoid the painful feelings.

"The first time I heard or saw abortion mentioned was when I got the hospital statements. The diagnosis and procedure said 'legal abortion.' When I read that it felt like I had been slapped across the face." Shelley

Will my medical insurance cover the procedure I choose?

Before you go any further it is important that you contact your insurance company, HMO, or doctor's office to find out what will be covered and what will not. Sometimes people spend days or weeks agonizing over the decision, then after they make it and the procedure is over, they receive a bill because it was not covered by their medical plan. Check this out as soon as possible.

What procedures are used to end a pregnancy?

This section deals with the methods of pregnancy termination used when a baby either has died or is still alive. It is by no means meant to replace the medical advice of your care provider. Rather it is meant to educate you about potential options as you work with your medical team attempting to make an informed decision that best fits your needs. Not all procedures may be available to you. You should discuss this carefully with your medical care provider. Use the material below to ask questions and find out what your options are.

When you are deciding which method you would prefer, you may want to find out if the baby is likely to be alive during the procedure or after

45

the birth. Discuss your wishes with your physician. Maybe you will want to hold and cradle your baby before death. Although it may seem hard to imagine, having some time with your baby alive and holding her/him during the last moments of life can become a very special, though painful, memory that you will cherish for the rest of your life.

Each physician and facility will have their own way of handling these procedures which are described here in a general way:

Induction of labor This procedure, which uses medication to artificially induce labor, is generally performed after the thirteenth week of pregnancy. You should expect it to be like real labor. You will experience contractions and will likely deliver vaginally unless there are other unusual circumstances that require a Caesarean section. You may be able to use medication to reduce the pain, since there is no worry about hurting the baby.

You will most likely be admitted to the Labor and Delivery floor at a hospital which is equipped to handle this procedure. After being settled into the room and having a history taken, you should inform the staff of any special things you want done during and after the delivery. Your partner may want to be present to offer support and be a part of this experience.

Prostaglandin may be administered via a vaginal suppository, or by an injection through the abdomen into the amniotic sac to begin uterine contractions. Occasionally other medications may be used to begin labor. A gel may be placed on the cervix to help it soften and dilate. Once the contractions start, labor usually lasts from 10 to 20 hours; however, it can be longer. The prostaglandin can produce uncomfortable symptoms such as fever, chills, nausea, diarrhea and other side effects.

When the contractions become stronger, additional medication can be given to make you more comfortable. *Ask for it if you feel you need pain relief.* The medications vary from IV pain killers to an epidural. The epidural procedure, performed by an anesthesiologist, relieves pain from the waist down. This enables you to be fully conscious, yet pain-free. It is important to note that many mothers regret being drugged too heavily with pain killers at the time of delivery because it makes their memories foggy and unclear.

"I had such a short time with my baby. Sadly, it was all so hazy because of the drugs that had been given to me. My memories are very important, especially years later since they are what ties me to my baby.

46

I wish they had discouraged the use of drugs instead of encouraging them." S

Once your baby is born, be sure to spend as much time with him/her as you wish. You may want to encourage the rest of your family to join you in sharing this precious time together. The section **Hello, Goodbye** will offer suggestions and more specifics. The **Appendix** has books and resources that can also be helpful to you.

"Having made our decision to terminate the pregnancy, my husband and I were given the option of which method we'd prefer. For me the decision was an easy one, induction and labor. I wanted a chance to hold my baby, to see him, feel him, smell him. I wanted him baptized and I wanted as many pictures of him as time would allow. Only one method, induction, could offer this to us. My husband was willing to support either decision I made since I was the one having to go through the physical procedure. I am so thankful we did it this way." Amy

"Holding our baby was the hardest thing for us, but we needed to see him and say hello. We had to tell him that we loved him and that we were sorry. Holding the baby gave us physical closure and helped us with starting to make an emotional closure." M.

"The biggest thing that I remember about being at the hospital was the feeling of adding punishment on top of punishment. Mercifully, I really experienced almost no pain. My baby just all of a sudden was born. I felt so numb. I hadn't taken any pain medication, but the length of time, along with the anti-nausea drugs and emotions of the day, had taken its toll. I remember everything, but just wasn't moved by it. I just sort of did what I had to do and let my husband do most of the talking. Thankfully, the night nurse let me sleep through the night and the next morning I was incredibly better. The first thing I did was to call family and friends, then I took a walk down to the nursery. Even though I knew I wouldn't be leaving the hospital with a baby, it was very comforting to me to see those babies. It was proof to me that most of the time pregnancy brings a happy ending: a normal, healthy baby." Gwen

Another advantage of induction of labor for pregnancy termination is that it allows a fetal evaluation, autopsy and genetic studies following delivery. Arriving at a correct diagnosis is pivotal to providing you with information about what happened, and the risks of recurrence in the future. This is the *only* time this critical information will be available to the medical team.

Dilation and Curettage (D & C) and Dilation and Evacuation (D & E) - These two procedures are sometimes used after miscarriages, especially when there is heavy bleeding. They are also used in therapeutic abortions. A D & C can be done up to about twelve week's gestation and a D & E up to about twenty weeks. Both procedures are usually relatively quick and, if medication is given, fairly pain-free. There is a minimal physical recovery period with these procedures.

In the D & C procedure, the cervix is dilated (opened) and a curettage is performed, in which the uterus is scraped of its contents. Pain relief may include a local anesthetic, a spinal, an epidural or general anesthesia. Oral medications for pain relief may also be prescribed.

The D & E procedure is used in patients whose pregnancy is more advanced. If it takes some time to schedule the procedure, the waiting time will not be easy, especially if the baby is kicking and feeling so alive.

Sometimes it can be difficult to find a nearby physician who is willing to perform this procedure. If you and your partner choose this method, your physician can refer you to a center where this procedure is performed, if it is not routinely done at your hospital. You might be referred to a special center such as an abortion clinic or a hospital that performs these procedures for pregnancy termination. You may find it difficult to be around teens and mothers who are aborting unwanted babies at these centers. In addition, the staff might not be used to comforting and caring for someone who is reluctantly terminating a wanted pregnancy. You may wish to talk with your doctor and the staff who will be doing the procedure before the appointment. Be a strong advocate for yourself in this setting.

Your partner may want to be in the room during the procedure. If watching what is happening is difficult for him, he may be able to stand or sit where he can hold your hand and look into your face. However, some facilities, especially abortion clinics, might not encourage or allow his presence. If this is important to you, discuss this before you schedule the procedure. They may be willing to bend the rules for you.

"We had almost a week to wait. At first I wanted to crawl into a hole and not come out until it was all over. I felt ashamed, embarrassed, and somehow freakish that this had happened to me. The waiting was indescribable! Whenever I saw my pregnant body in the mirror, I felt like throwing up. I could still feel the baby kicking during those six

days between getting the results and having the abortion. It was just agony! And now I could take any medications I wanted; after all, I'd be killing this fetus in a few days, so it didn't matter. It was a horrible switch, to go from being careful and protective of this new life to deciding to end it." Rose (Green 1992)

The D & E is usually a two-day process. On the first day, dilataria or laminaria are inserted into the cervix to dilate it. These are tiny sticks which expand when they come in contact with moisture. As they expand, they dilate the cervix. This is relatively painless and you can usually go about your daily activities while they are in place, though it is normal for mild cramping to occur. The following day at the clinic or hospital, a form of pain relief is given, either local anesthetic, a spinal, an epidural or general anesthesia. Then vacuum suction is used to extract the contents of the uterus. After the procedure you may feel groggy from the anesthetic. Otherwise, there should be very little discomfort from the procedure. With any of the procedures there will be bleeding afterwards. This should be very much like a menstrual period, heavier the first few days and tapering off as the days go by.

Because the baby's body and the pregnancy tissue will be broken up during the procedure, an autopsy cannot be done. The information from an autopsy might have helped determine the presence of structural abnormalities or lead to a specific diagnosis. However, you can still ask for chromosome studies to be done to look for abnormalities and the gender of the baby. You may also want to ask for any other possible tests that can be done.

Holding and seeing the remains of your baby following the D & C or D & E is possible, but it won't be the whole baby you had hoped for. You may ask to look at your baby's remains or receive his or her ashes if you wish. This can serve as a means of saying goodbye and may allow you to face the reality of what has happened and, in time, move ahead. If you do not wish to view the remains of the pregnancy and baby there are other ways to memorialize your baby, such as through an ultrasound picture, memories of your pregnancy and little mementos that you can make or buy in honor of your child. Some parents admit to feeling a detachment, or having confused feelings, similar to mothers who miscarry without a body to look at and few concrete memories. Be open to the idea of finding ways to help make your baby real. If you loved this baby, you probably won't get over this by pretending nothing happened. This subject is covered more in depth in the section **What are my options after the pregnancy is ended?**

"I couldn't face the fact of having to go through labor, but the hardest part of the D & E was knowing that my baby was being dismembered. I still have trouble thinking about that." Dorothy

"Due to the procedure used to terminate the pregnancy, I did not get to see or hold my baby. While it was medically necessary and I understand the reasons for it, I have always regretted that I didn't get a chance to physically see and hold my baby. My husband and I did a number of things to help ourselves through the aftermath. We had the body of the baby cremated and his remains placed in a lovely brass jewelry box, which was then sealed. It is kept in our room. " Susan

"Although my husband and I were 'comfortable' with our choice to have the D & E procedure, I was not prepared for such a black and white experience. I went into the procedure awake and carrying my baby within. Then I awoke in recovery with the realization that our sweet little girl had been taken from my body." Holli

Hormonal changes should be anticipated following pregnancy termination, since hormone levels were elevated during pregnancy and are now normalizing. Some of the things you may experience are: cramping, fatigue, crying spells, mood swings, night sweats, chills, hot flashes and increased perspiration and urination. Your milk may even come in, thus it will be important to learn about how to handle this occurrence. In addition, the common responses of grief after loss can lead to intense feelings. Your caregiver may have some ideas on how to cope, including suggesting medication that might be helpful.

"I wish someone had told me about the importance of binding my breasts; even a very tight bra would have helped. Apparently every movement of the body, even walking, is a stimulant to the breasts to produce milk unless they are bound. It was horrible and I wish I would have been able to do something to avoid or lessen it. Anyone who has a miscarriage, a termination or an infant death should discuss this with their doctor ahead of time." Debra

Be sure to follow the hygiene, medication and activity recommendations that your medical team has suggested. As always, if you have any questions, be sure to call and ask them.

Dad, you might feel somewhat left out during this time. So much is happening to your partner and there is so little you can do. However, your presence and support is extremely important to her. And needless to say, her well-being is most likely your major concern at this time.

But do take into account some of *your* needs, too. Share your thoughts, your feelings and your hugs. Acknowledge your own grief.

"Overall, the induction was more painful and more like a full-term delivery than I had expected, so it was very, very helpful to have my husband there holding my hand. Even though there is a lot of waiting around for the dads, I hope they know how much they are needed." Debra

"While it was hard to be there, watching Susan suffer, I was glad I could see our baby born and that I was with Susan at a very important and painful time. Only later, much later, was I able to begin to face my grief. At the time, my wife and child were my first concerns." Greg

If you do get autopsy results after any of these procedures it is possible that you will receive confirmation of the problem, which may serve to ease your mind. However, in some cases, even after the autopsy and genetic studies there exists some uncertainty about what happened. You might also learn that your baby only had some of the spectrum of problems possible, based on the prenatal diagnosis. There is no guarantee that every one of today's tests and technologies can give accurate and complete answers. If you are surprised and/or upset by the results, seek support. More information can also be helpful along with speaking to a genetic counselor if you haven't already done so.

"The autopsy results reassured me that I made the right decision. They also told me that the results showed no more of a chance for it to happen to me again than to anyone else. This was a relief." Dorothy

"We were very upset when we learned that while our baby did, indeed, have spina bifida, the degree of severity was less than we expected. This caused us to wonder what her life could have been like if we hadn't terminated the pregnancy. This is something we are learning to live with. It hasn't been easy; we have been seeing a counselor and have talked extensively with our doctor. It really was a chance we took when we made the decision." P.

What are my options after the pregnancy is ended?

While there is no "best thing" to do, there are many options. During the past decade bereaved parents have expressed a strong desire (or deep regrets if they didn't get to do these things) to see, hold, examine and be with their baby for awhile. The need to "say hello" seems important in order to get ready to "say goodbye." The section **Hello, Goodbye** goes into more detail about how and why to do this. For further

51

details, books such as *Empty Arms* and *Hello Means Goodbye* are written specifically about how to say "hello," create memories, include other family members and what to expect in the days and months to come. It would take a whole book to prepare you for this very special time, thus if you want more specifics you may want to turn to a short, readable book such as this one.

"I had labor induced. I was terrified the entire 12 hours. I was afraid for myself and I was afraid of what I would see and how I would act. It was horrible. The unknown always is. The delivery itself was difficult to handle. Yet, I envisioned my deceased Grandmother and several close friends reaching out their arms for the baby. I felt he was being cared for. This was helpful. We held the baby, named him, talked to him, unwrapped and examined him. I had cross-stitched a note, from us to the baby, on the blanket he was buried with. " J.

You may be reluctant at first to see your baby, thinking that it will be better for you for you not to. While there surely are people who are at peace with not seeing their baby, most families who have not seen their baby talk of their regrets. They felt robbed of this important time to meet their child and create the memories that would sustain them over time.

"I was in complete denial. We didn't want anything to do with the baby. I didn't want to even know the sex of the child I was going to deliver. This was wrong! As much time as possible should be spent with the baby. And strong emotional counseling should be sought out **before** *delivery, if possible."* Jackie

"I didn't see my baby because at the time it seemed to be the best decision. I think that others facing this decision need to know how important it is to at least see their child to enable them to say goodbye. I wish I had." Shelley

As hard as it may be to look at and experience your baby, spend time showering your love on your baby. This is your one chance. Dress and undress him or her, bathe and have pictures taken of you holding your baby, if you wish. You will cherish these in the future. They will be the memories and mementos that will bring you through the more difficult times. Maybe you can learn the sex of the baby, although that is not always possible. Naming your baby can sometimes be helpful to make him/her seem more real to you and others. Naming can further legitimize that you really had a baby, not just tissue, a miscarriage or an abortion.

If you desire a religious ceremony, talk with your clergy about a baptism or blessing ceremony. You may want to encourage your other children, and relatives, to see the baby, too, and spend some time with him or her. You can do any of these things, some of them or none of them. Just be aware that avoiding the hard, short-term pain of spending time with your baby could be replaced by long-term pain and regrets. You can't avoid the pain, so look within your heart to see what you want and need to do now.

"We held Michael and took pictures and also had him baptized. My husband, parents and my sister and grandmother were also there and held him. I was in such shock and also on so much medication. I wish that I would have done more! I wish now that we would have spent more time alone with him and not felt so rushed." S.

How do I deal with my faith and/or guilt?

If your faith is such that you feel guilty about your decision, you will want to face this at some point. Or maybe you have concerns about God, His role, your faith values along with other spiritual issues. Talk with a pastoral advisor to explore your feelings, your faith and God's forgiveness. Write down your questions and concerns. Talk with others who might help you. Use your coping skills. Remember prayer and meditation are tools for healing and forgiveness.

"My pastor shared some helpful things with us:
*• That if we all prayed to God for guidance and came to a unanimous agreement, peace could be attained. This was not to imply that we would feel **good** about the decision, but that we would make peace with God and ourselves.*
• That the prenatal testing that is available today was not available when God walked the earth and when the Bible was written, and because of this our specific issue could not be addressed in the Bible. The Bible is not a scientific journal. Our God is aware of the times and of the tools that we have and knows why we make the decisions that we do.
• People can only make me feel guilty if I let them." Gwen

Difficult choices are made out of love. The decision to terminate has painful consequences, but may have been the better choice for you. Use prayer to speak with your God. If you desire forgiveness seek it. If you are angry share it.

How do I tell people?

You have ended the pregnancy and may be afraid that others will judge you or make some comment that will hurt or embarrass you. Abortion is such an emotionally laden topic in our present-day society. Some people are passionate in their beliefs about abortion, sometimes no matter what the special circumstances are. You may have even shared similar beliefs. But until they are in your situation, they will never know the agony of facing such a decision. Whatever their reasons, religious, moral or otherwise, people may make remarks that feel hurtful. You will need to think of ways to handle these comments. Try not to take this personally. Don't let others' comments hurt you or make you feel guilty. Resist this! Although you don't need to rationalize your decision to them, their comments may cause you to re-examine what has happened at times. Be prepared that this is normal. Don't use all your energy trying to make others understand and/or change their judgments. You need all the energy now to grieve and go on.

Now that the birth is over, hopefully you will come to the only conclusion that really matters to you now, *this was the best option you had at the time*. Nothing can change that, and now you must and will go on from here. It may be hard to tolerate the remarks of others when you are so emotionally devastated, but in time, it becomes easier.

"I very rarely use the word 'abortion.' I usually say 'Jonathon's death.'" E.

You will need to decide how much you want to share with family and friends what has happened. What do you want to tell people? How will you tell them, and who do you tell?

There is no magic formula or answer about *how* to tell people. The answer will have to come from within you. Take a good look at your need for support and open communication as you think about the likely response of your family and friends. There is no way to predict how each person will respond to your news.

You may be confused about who to tell and how much to share. If you think that some people will be able to handle this but others might not, you can choose to limit who you tell. Of course, you run the risk that others will find out. If people are judgmental and don't understand, you may choose to share only that your baby died. If you keep it a secret from everyone, however, you may isolate yourself and make it difficult to get support at least from those who would understand and be sensitive. On the other hand, you may choose to be open and honest with many people or even everyone about your decision. Sharing your experience with others is a valid method of coping and can be an important part of the healing process. You will need to make these decisions based on your experience and your good judgment.

"I chose to tell only a few friends and two family members the truth. The others thought it was a miscarriage. I felt I had to do it that way, but it has been a very isolated grief because of this." Dorothy

"We told very few people before we terminated. We had enough to get through without added suggestions and advice. Afterwards, we placed an obituary notice in the local papers. This let people know the baby had died, but eliminated the majority of questions and explanations." J.

"We told a few people the truth. The loneliness of keeping the truth from so many adds anguish to an already painful experience." E.

"I find that it's not always necessary to tell people how the pregnancy ended. I sometimes just say, 'She was born at 20 weeks and did not survive.'" Debra

"I found myself feeling angry at those I had to 'walk' through awkward conversations. I wished they could have just sent a card. I also found more comfort from those people who merely expressed, 'I'm sorry' or 'I don't know what to say,' than from those who felt the need to say 'It just wasn't meant to be' or 'At least you found out now instead of later.'" Holli

"We sent out a birth/death announcement when we terminated our pregnancy. We wrote a poem about our daughter, put her name on the announcement, and mailed it to those people who we were close to. It was a concrete way to acknowledge her as a real person and a member of our family." Sheila

"I told a few close friends the 'whole' story. I have not heard back from some of them since. Be prepared—it is cruel, but some people simply cannot accept your decision. This hurts tremendously, but it is their problem, not yours. We all make our own choices. Now we say the baby had a severe congenital defect and was stillborn. I do not have the energy or desire to defend my decision to anyone who doesn't feel the same way. It is not up for debate." J.

Sometimes I feel I am going crazy.

Once you get home you may experience an overwhelming feeling of emptiness. Some describe it as a "big dark hole," a frightening and lonely place. You no longer have the excitement of a due date to wait for. Instead, you may dread that day. Understandably, you may feel there is *nothing* to look forward to. Things have changed so quickly and drastically. Perhaps only a few days ago you were pregnant and expecting to share your future with this special, loved child. You are no longer pregnant or a family expecting a baby. *"Who am I ?"* you may ask!

Anger is one of the most common feelings parents have after such an experience. You may feel anger at the medical world, your doctor, God, your partner and even your baby. You may be filled with emptiness, sadness, confusion or a sense of hopelessness. Shame, fear, regrets and feelings of failure are other strong emotions that some people experience. You may feel failure because your baby is not perfect, or because you are not the perfect parents you hoped you would be. It might help just to know these are normal feelings. They are so human, yet sometimes difficult to admit and express. Their intensity may be frightening and unexpected. This is also normal.

You may experience guilt or a sense of responsibility. Each day many of us may feel guilt and shame for things in our lives. We have regrets over things we "should have" or "wish we would have" done. Significant events, like the death of a baby, may cause an intensity of guilt feelings. They may haunt us. You may want to discuss these feelings with people who are sensitive and who understand. Sharing can sometimes lessen the pain. You may find it helpful to talk with a clergyperson, counselor, your partner, a relative or a friend. Write your feelings down, and most of all, if you do feel some guilt, work on forgiving and letting go. Sometimes the physical release of exercise is helpful in these situations.

There is no predictable pattern or set of feelings that are common to everyone. In addition, no one can free you of these feelings. Talk or write about them, find ways to express and release them. If they are not expressed and shared in some way they can cause physical and emotional harm. Work on accepting that these feelings are part of your love and the pain you feel because of your loss. Have hope that you will heal.

It is also normal if you *don't* have these feelings. You may not feel guilt, and that can sometimes lead to confusion. Maybe you pick up clues from others that you *should* feel guilty, yet you may have found some peace and acceptance among the many other emotions you are feeling. It's okay if guilt is not one of them.

"A lot of my confusion stemmed from the vast difference between what I was feeling and the message I was getting from everyone else. I felt very deeply about our loss but it seemed that most people said light things like, 'Oh well, try again.' Reading books like **Empty Arms** *and talking with understanding friends helped validate my feelings. I still sometimes feel that I have to fight for the right to grieve for this baby...What has helped me the most has been writing down my feelings—not the medical facts, but my feelings—good and bad. I realize now that we did make a caring, loving decision for Christina."*
Debra

"At first I told myself that since my husband and I did not **doubt** *our decision to terminate this pregnancy, emotionally the abortion would be the same as a miscarriage, and in fact a miscarriage might be worse if you didn't know the cause and didn't know what was wrong with your baby. While this last point is probably true enough, it's not the* **whole** *truth. I have had to face the fact that we* **chose** *to kill this fetus, which we had conceived in love and hope. I have had to face the fact that I felt the baby kicking as I walked into the abortion clinic. I have had to face images of blood and death, and of a fetus in pieces...this is difficult for me to write...but I must be honest. I cried and cried and cried about this. It comes down to facing and accepting responsibility for the abortion, and for our decision to abort. Note I say 'responsibility,' not 'guilt.' Guilt would imply that I had done something wrong, or made a choice which I now regret. 'Responsibility,' on the other hand, means that I recognize that I did make the choice and that I can stand up and accept that choice." Rose (Green 1992)*

"The guilt was overwhelming. I was angry! I hated the doctors, the nurses, my pastor...Was I so selfish a mother that I chose to end my baby's life 3 months before it would have ended naturally? Did I spare him a horrible death or did I rob him of a few more weeks of warmth and love in my womb? I was devastated. It was my fault. I was crying all the time. Finally a friend told me about a counselor and I went to see her. She said I hadn't grieved for the baby. She advised me to get as many mementos and information on the baby as possible. Eventually these things helped me." Jackie

"A chaplain spoke at a support group on guilt. He made statements indicating that the damage done from a decision like this is for some people irreparable and that we may never be able to rid ourselves of the

guilt. *He further spoke about us living in a society that wants us to live free from guilt, and that he doesn't necessarily agree that we **should** be released from all guilt. This made me feel guilty about **not** feeling guilty. I also do not believe that a person should be able to go through life without the burden of guilt. But I don't believe that God, or my baby, would want us to feel such guilt. We've suffered enough."*
Gwen

Searching for a reason

You may feel that if you can just find a reason for your tragedy, you won't let yourself be hurt like this again or you might better understand it. Searching for a cause or reason for your misfortune is normal. It's hard to feel so vulnerable and out of control. You may resist the idea that things just happen and search hard for a cause, thus trying to regain some control. You may want someone or something to be responsible. You may torment yourself thinking "if only," "I should have" or "I shouldn't have." However, you will want to remember that you would not have intentionally harmed your unborn child. These problems were not *caused* by you, or God or anyone else. They often happen as accidents of nature.

"The best day for relieving guilt was the day of my post-partum checkup and autopsy report. The suspected problems were confirmed along with other problems. When the doctor stated that I did nothing to cause the problems nor could I have done anything to prevent them, it really hit home. Others had told me this but I didn't believe them. I felt they were trying to relieve me from suffering from guilt. How could they know? I believed my doctor." Gwen

FAMILY, FRIENDS AND OTHERS

Getting support from others

As you share your story with others, be prepared for many different reactions. People will struggle with what to say, how to react and how to help you. Many may offer advice, question the diagnosis and the medical care you have been given, or even say things that minimize your tragedy. Some may appear harsh or insensitive, while others cry with you and show empathy. This is a tense time for your relatives, co-workers and friends. They suffer for you, for your baby and for themselves. Do not try to take care of them. Take care of yourself and allow others to care for you, as hard as this may be.

It cannot be emphasized enough that everyone needs to find someone with whom they can share their pain. In addition to your partner, you will need someone you can be truthful with; someone who will not judge you, but who will support you and help you feel safe. That person may be a friend, relative, clergyperson, counselor or someone who has shared a similar experience. Express and release your troubling thoughts. Tell them what might be helpful to you. People will take their cues from you, often waiting and saying nothing until they learn what you want and need. This support can help to replenish you at an overwhelming time and add strength to your relationship with your partner. Keep the communication channels open between you and your partner, as well as with your support system.

"A close friend is invaluable and was one of my greatest sources of help. You may find it surprising who will come to your aid. Even my in-laws who are anti-abortion were very supportive." Susan

"Many of my co-workers, mostly men, were very supportive of me when they learned there was something wrong with the baby. They really wanted to know what was happening, they expressed genuine interest and care. Many shared their own personal stories, even people I barely knew. Some men sent us notes that they were praying for us. I felt truly supported by my co-workers at the auto plant." Bob

A support group may be a safe place where you may share your grief and agony, your hopes and fears with other people who understand. There are hundreds of groups around the country for families whose baby has died and many other groups for families raising a child who has disabilities. Unfortunately, there are at this time few groups for people who have had to make the difficult decision to terminate a pregnancy. Talk with support group facilitators *before* attending a meeting to learn how your needs would be met by a particular group. Maybe you could be connected with someone who has experienced a similar loss, even if you never go to the group.

It can be hard getting yourself to that first support group meeting, especially if you don't know someone else who is going. It takes some people many months before they are ready to attend a meeting, while others are able to go shortly after their baby's death. You might find it helpful to bring your partner, a friend or relative to the first meeting.

You may need to find additional means to deal with your pain and grief. Writing in a journal, writing a letter to your baby or to God are some ways to get your feelings out. These writings may be invaluable in the coming days as you look back and see how far you have come in the grieving process. You may also find other outlets such as: exercise, woodworking, weaving, sculpting, painting, needlework, music, dance, drawing and physical activity.

My care providers don't seem to understand my feelings.

It has been only in the last decade or so that science has provided us with the technology to diagnose so many problems early in pregnancy. Our social systems for dealing with this technology trail behind, however. Few members of the clergy, for example, have had formal training in providing for those who, like you, face such difficult decisions. This dilemma may not have been addressed when counselors and psychologists were trained. Medical students may have learned about the medical side of it, but not necessarily the emotional side. Those who have learned probably learned from experience. You may find a good ally in genetic counselors, who have both training and experience in prenatal diagnosis counseling, decision making, and providing support after pregnancy loss.

No one really knows exactly how to help you the most at this time. Professionals who care about you may not always be able to offer you what you truly need. Doctors, clergy or even counselors cannot feel what you feel, unless they have also faced a similar dilemma. Even then, they cannot know what you feel or want. They hurt for you and wish to help, so try to be understanding and open with them. Tell them what you need from them. As hard as this may be, it is the only way they will really learn how to support you and others.

"I was pregnant. I had a baby who was alive and is now dead. Yet both my minister and doctor act as if it were just a minor event. Maybe if I would have named her and had a funeral they would treat me like the mother that I am." E.

How do we tell our children?

Including your other living children is imperative, yet it may not be easy due to the stress you are under. Tell the truth, or at least as much of the truth as you can. How much you will be able to tell them will be dependent on their ages, whether or not they knew about this pregnancy, and your own comfort level. Don't think that by avoiding the topic it will go away in their minds. It won't. They already know that something serious is going on. They can tell by what you say, what you don't say and the atmosphere around the house. They may feel they were somehow at fault, that their secret wishes or behavior caused this. Make sure they understand it wasn't their fault. Many times children take responsibility for problems happening around them, which is a way for them to explain or understand it. The general rule followed by most child development experts is to talk openly about what is happening. Silence and secrets can be very damaging to families over time. Instead of secrets, be open and honest.

"From the start we were completely open and honest with our almost four-year-old son, Joe. During the 17 weeks of waiting we talked about death, how very very sick the baby was, that it was nobody's fault, etc. We included Joe in most of our tears and decisions. We read books on life and death, we left the door open for questions and tears in the months/years ahead. He decided to see his brother at the hospital. He gave him a special toy and placed it in his casket. He attended the funeral and continues to visit the grave. " Cubby

"Because the baby's prognosis was so poor it seemed everyone had given up hope for the baby. With tears of sadness we explained this to our daughter, Emily, who then said, 'I don't want to be sad, I want to be happy. The baby's going to get better, probably on Tuesday.' We then realized that she was the only one who hadn't given up hope." Bob

Anticipate that it may take children many conversations and lots of time to really understand that the baby has died or has severe problems. Be patient and be prepared to answer their questions over and over again. The questions will change over the years as their awareness and understanding grows and as they continue to grow and develop.

*"We told our children that the baby was very sick and that momma was going to the hospital. Then we told them the baby was so sick that it died. Now that we know the details, we told them it was a boy and the doctors found out just how sick he really was, how **not** normal he was. When they are older and can better understand we will tell them of our decision."* M.

If you continue the pregnancy you could choose to say you are worried about the baby, that s/he might be born with some problems or you could drop little hints while you wait.

Using examples taken from nature can sometimes help children understand. The case of the egg that never hatches, the puppy without an ear, the kitten who dies at birth, or the young tree that splits and dies after a storm illustrate that it is common for things to go wrong in this world without blame or explanation.

Sheila told her children, ages three and seven, by using this metaphor: *"When cookies are made the baker puts in eggs and sugar, a whole lot of flour, a tiny bit of salt and some chocolate chips. Then it's mixed together and baked and you get cookies. What do you think would happen if a tiny pinch of salt was left out? You would probably hardly notice something was missing, would you? Now what do you think would happen if chocolate chips were left out? Well, you would still have cookies, but they wouldn't be exactly what you had planned. You would still be able to eat them, they would still be delicious, but they wouldn't be what you initially thought you wanted. Now imagine that someone forgot to put in the flour. Flour is the most important ingredient of the cookie. Without flour you really don't have cookies. If you tried to bake them this way it really wouldn't work. You just would never end up with cookies if you didn't put in the flour.*

"Well, our baby was a little bit like that. If our baby was just missing maybe a toe or a finger, we would hardly be able to tell that something was missing. We would still have a wonderful baby who could do the things babies are supposed to do. If our baby was a boy instead of the girl we had hoped for, we would still have a wonderful baby that we could play with. We would have loved that baby no matter what it was—once it was a member of our family. However, sometimes more serious things can go wrong when a baby is being made. We don't always know why. If the most important parts are missing, like the flour in the cookies, then we won't have the healthy, whole baby that we had hoped for. Our baby was like that. Something went wrong when she was being put together and unfortunately some of the most

important parts were missing. We would not have had the healthy baby we had hoped for. I am so sorry that this baby will not be able to live with us. But she will always be a special member of our family and we will never forget her. She will live up in heaven with God and Auntie Trish."

Using this type of story with children may help them to better understand that the baby was not healthy and could not live a normal life. Children will always ask questions, usually the ones you have not prepared for. Count on that. Try to answer their questions honestly, using terms they can relate to. When they are old enough to understand you will want to decide if you wish to share what actually happened. If your child has already been told some of the truth, this further explanation will just be an evolution of the story.

Children, much like adults, try to explain away such shocking events by looking at their own behaviors and beliefs. They may fear that their thoughts, wishes or complaints caused this to happen. They may wonder if this is their punishment. They may also fear that if something bad happens to them you may have to make a similar decision about their life. Help them to understand that neither they, nor you, nor the doctors caused or could prevent what happened. Questions may come up often and may need to be discussed through the coming years. In addition, they may have fears of their own death or yours. They may have trouble sleeping or fear getting sick.

"When we explained Lisa's death to Amy and Brett, we told them Lisa was missing some body parts and some were not working correctly. We thought it most important to emphasize that Brett, Amy, Mom and Dad were not missing parts and our bodies worked correctly, to minimize their fears." Barb

There are a number of excellent books written on grief and loss for children. *How Do We Tell the Children, Lifetimes, The Tenth Good Thing About Barney, Thumpy's Story* and *The Fall of Freddy the Leaf* are good books you might find helpful. See the **Appendix** for information on these books. For more recommendations check your library and your local mental health centers, churches and funeral homes.

63

HELLO, GOODBYE

Making memories—why is this important?

No matter how your child died, you will need to say your *goodbyes* in a meaningful way. Rituals and ceremonies are important in the grieving and healing process. They are a way for us to express our love. However, before you rush into those goodbyes be sure you spend some time saying *hello,* taking time to meet and experience your baby. They both become the memories that will heal you over time. Unlike an older child or adult whose life brought many memories, you have only dreams of your baby. Now can be the time when you take it slowly— hold your baby, bathe and dress him or her, sharing this experience with close family and friends as you create out of these moments the memories you will cherish for a lifetime.

"We had a natural childbirth. My being awake gave us the opportunity to be included 100 percent in the birth of our son. He was baptized and given to us immediately after birth. He looked perfect and beautiful to us. We spent the next few hours with Frank. We held, bathed, and dressed him. We clipped a lock of his hair and loved him with all our hearts. Our son, Joe, came to see him also." Cubby

"We have a special packet of memories that is kept in the cedar chest— photos, hat, tape measure, baptismal shell, etc. I also wrote the story of our son and put it with the packet. Once I wrote the story and the details were on paper I felt better. I needed to write down the details, since the fear of forgetting worried me." Mary

Read books/booklets on helping you say hello and goodbye to your baby who has died or will die. This type of planning may not be easy but, as one mother suggested, doing these very painful things were the medicine to heal her broken heart. The **Appendix** lists books to help you plan this time carefully.

What are my rights and options in caring for my baby's body?

Each state varies in its laws as to your rights and the requirements for caring for your baby's body. Whether your baby is considered miscarried, aborted, stillborn or an infant death you should have the right to decide if you want testing or not, unless there is a communicable disease or reason for the medical examiner to authorize testing. You also should have the right to be in charge of whether you have a funeral, memorial service and/or cremation. Depending on your state and local requirements you may or may not have to use a funeral director to bury your baby. Often babies under 20 to 22 weeks do not require as much paperwork as older babies and few laws exist that govern their final disposition, although burying a baby on your property may be illegal in your city or county. While cost may be the main reason you might choose to take care of making all the arrangements for your baby, don't jump to the conclusion that a funeral director's services will be costly. Before you decide, check out your options and the prices. Funeral directors offer an invaluable service and usually can give much assistance at a trying time, as well as share resources and make referrals for coping in the days that follow.

If you want to take your baby's remains to another state, check with a funeral director about how to do this. You may need some paperwork filled out. The hospital might not be accustomed to these requests, especially for smaller babies which they may view as lab tissue and not a baby. The hospital may have rules about options for caring for your baby's remains, but it is your baby, so learn what your rights are and let them know what you want to do. Let them know your desires. You could ask your doctor, one of the nurses, call the hospital administrator, an attorney or the Department of Health if you need assistance understanding your rights or getting what you need.

DIFFICULT DAYS

My days are up and down. When will I feel whole and happy again?

There will be depressing times, lonely times and, amazingly enough, good times in the days ahead. The good times may be few and far between at first, but they will come. Some people say that the days seem to get darker in the beginning, once the shock has worn off and people have stopped inquiring about how you are doing and offering help. This is all normal, though it may seem disturbing to you. Be sure you find a good support network; maybe relatives, friends, a pastoral counselor, a support group or another parent who has gone through something similar.

Many who have suffered a loss such as yours report feeling the baby kick or hearing the baby cry. Rest assured that other mothers have experienced these feelings. Mom or Dad, you might want to sleep all the time or not at all. You could also have some or many of the following feelings: a tightness in your chest, difficulty breathing, disinterest in food, or overeating to fill the emptiness, tiredness, and/or an inability to get out of bed or participate in normal activities. You may feel envious and jealous of others who have healthy babies. Your arms may physically ache. You may bury yourself in work or a project so you don't have to think. You may want another child very badly or may feel so afraid that you don't want to even think about attempting another pregnancy. It is different for each person, but you will find that most of these reactions are considered usual grief responses. While most feelings including some depression are normal and a necessary part of grieving, be aware that frequent thoughts about giving up on life or hurting someone is a sign that you need help. **If you think you might hurt yourself or someone else immediately seek help from a crisis hotline, your physician or a counselor .**

Dad, you will find that people inquire about your partner but often forget to ask how you are doing. They will assume that you don't hurt as much as she does or that you have completely recovered. *You* know that is not true. It's impossible to compare the amount of hurt one feels with another. It may be that you are offering your her strength now and putting your pain aside until later. Many men describe feeling that they could only begin to grieve once they knew their partner was going to be all right. Many men say they cry on the way to work, in the shower or while by themselves. In our society, men are often expected to be "strong" and "in control." Expressing emotions, especially sadness and sorrow, is often discouraged. Instead of following this pattern of "swallowing" emotions, you may find it helpful to release your emotions through physical activity, writing, discussions or other outlets that seem appropriate.

If you are in the process of giving your baby up for adoption or have already done so, you may feel as though you have suffered a death, yet you know the baby's life continues. Whether or not you will be able to have contact with the adopting family will be up to you, them and the adoption agency. You may feel better if you stay in contact with the family, or you might choose not to. Trust your feelings and find others to talk with about this. This will not be an easy time. You love this baby and want the best for him or her. You have decided that another loving family could offer a better life to your baby. Your decision was a great and loving gift and sacrifice. Accept this and realize you are not a failure. Rather, it took courage to be realistic about your limitations.

If your baby lives and has problems, naturally you will still grieve for the healthy baby you wanted and hoped for. You may be physically or emotionally exhausted from the care you must provide. This is normal, but it doesn't make it any easier. You may have trouble finding time for yourself and often feel overwhelmed. The strain may be felt by other family members. Your children, who see all the attention going to this baby, may feel cheated. Alternative caretakers, even on an occasional basis, will be important for you. Much of what you do each day will be to survive and hope. You will still need lots of support, and medical, emotional and spiritual care in the days and years ahead. Use your local resources, neighbors and family to aid you during the difficult times. Call your social service agency and doctor to locate support and information. Your needs will change over time as your baby grows. It's likely that you will find many days of joy, beauty and love in your child's life. Remember those times during the low moments.

"I have learned to accept the cards that I am dealt. Jeremy has enriched our lives more than I could have ever imagined. While we feel bad for him at times, for the things that may be hard or impossible for him to do, he seems so happy and well adjusted. We are thankful that he is with us, a living member of our family." K.

Despite your knowing that you made the best decision you could at the time, there will be questions, regrets and "what ifs." You can't go back, you can only go on. Don't second-guess yourself. Look ahead and try to be positive about life. Trust in your ability to handle problems as they arise, ask for help when you need it and believe in yourself! Your attitude will go a long way in helping the situation.

I have fantasies and dreams, some very disturbing.

Dreaming is a very natural occurrence. It can be a way of putting things right, or working through tough situations and gaining some perspective and peace. Not all dreams or fantasies are pleasant or helpful at the time. Sometimes they can be quite disturbing and awaken you from sleep. Nightmares may make you afraid to sleep at all You may want to share these dreams with someone, write them down, or try to put the disturbing ones out of your mind, until you are able to deal with them. It might be helpful to find a dream book at your bookstore or library. Seek help from a counselor if they become intolerable.

"I am tormented by fantasies and weird ideas that come and go...In one fantasy I have been offered the choice that if I give up my baby, my infertile sister will get pregnant and will have a healthy, normal baby. I consent because it is worth losing our baby so my sister can have one...Also, I keep replaying the phone call scene the way it should have been...I fantasize, too, that we decided not to believe the results and to continue the pregnancy....In the first weeks I was tormented by the fear that the lab had made an error..." Rose (Green 1992)

My emotions are sometimes more intense than I think they should be.

Bereavement and mourning cannot be predicted or controlled. It helps if you understand that it's natural to have many emotions at this time and in the days ahead. You may cry a lot, keep to yourself, focus on work to stay busy or lack concentration, feel angry and powerless, be listless and depressed and much more. There is no set formula or timeline for feelings. They come and go at will, it seems. It is not always possible to control them, no matter how hard you try.

"I should be feeling better by now, yet I am often overcome by sadness, sorrow and anger. Sometimes it seems my feelings are more intense than when she first died. Thankfully, I have met others in a similar situation and they tell me they can relate to these feelings. It helps not to be the only one. Maybe I'm not going crazy after all." K.

Do men and women grieve differently?

Be aware that often men and women grieve differently. All people grieve in a uniquely personal way and how we grieve also varies from one culture to another. Typically, but not always, women may have a greater need to talk and will more openly express their feelings. They may have a need to be creative or to turn their tragedy into helping others. Many men usually do not share their personal feelings as openly. It is common for men to keep their grief inside, to look forward, not backward. For some, physical activity or projects may be a healthy outlet. Whenever there are differences, no matter what they are, they can cause added strain and misunderstanding between partners. Some people may resent their partner because they feel as if they are *not* grieving. This misreading of their feelings adds to the problem. Many partners have asked their partner not to go to a support group or look at the pictures of the baby so much because it makes their partner sad. There are many ways of coping. Both partners need to realize they will probably grieve very differently and they need to be understanding of these differences. Keep communication lines open, and seek support from others in addition to each other.

"I often found it difficult to concentrate and keep my mind on my work. I was thinking about the baby and Lynn a lot." Russ

Many couples believe that the crisis brought them closer together and helped their relationship become stronger. Others find themselves disagreeing often and have ongoing problems in their relationship. Be careful not to let this loss bring about another loss—that of your partner and your relationship. Seek help from a third party; a counselor, pastoral advisor or trusted professional if you are experiencing problems communicating or relating. It is better to get help now, before it is too late.

My faith carries me through at times and at other times I feel deserted.

The familiar story of the "Footprints" may be something you can relate to at this time. The anguishing person asks where Jesus was when he needed Him. After all wasn't there only one pair of footprints in the sand during the hardest parts of life's journey? Jesus' reply was that during those dark days, "I carried you." Maybe you, too, feel at times that you have been deserted or even betrayed. If your faith has been important to you or is important now, try to talk and pray about this. Do not just give up, thinking that you have been abandoned. It is normal and healthy to be angry with God. He can handle your anger. Some people believe strongly that God is crying with you and feels your pain. Talk with a pastor, rabbi, lay minister, relative or friend about your struggles now. It's okay to question your faith or God's role. You have just been through a very traumatic experience. Yet, seek the support, when you are able.

"I have gained some peace and comfort through prayer and writing letters to God. My anger with God doesn't surface as often anymore. But I know its okay to feel that anger when it comes." E.

*"I always thought I could not, would not, **ever** be able to abort a child. When faced with this decision, my first reaction was total shock and disbelief. I was **afraid** that I wouldn't be able to handle it. I was **ashamed** that I felt afraid and I was **frightened**. I was only able to resolve this anguish through reading, talking with my chaplain, writing letters and confessing my sins to God. Only then did I feel at peace with myself, only after I was able to admit my feelings of guilt and anger, even though I knew we made the right decision and had no regrets, only sadness for our baby and myself. But as a Christian and a firm believer in "reverence for all life" I had to somehow realize, accept and forgive myself for what I felt was wrong, in spite of everything. And I accepted God's grace after I asked Him for forgiveness."* J.

Some people find their faith strengthens in crisis. They turn to God in prayer and meditation and feel His love which helps them get through the long days and the difficult nights. Maybe you feel that without your faith you wouldn't have made it this far. You rely on God and your spirituality to endure and cope. Continue to build on your faith and share it with others in your family, such as your children, who may be hurting.

Due dates, anniversaries and holidays

Special days such as a due date, an anniversary or other holidays can become bittersweet, especially if your baby has died. The due date often becomes a date that remains in your mind for a long time. Whether your baby died or was born early, this day will likely hold extra meaning for you. You may still be recovering from the shock of what has happened. Future due dates will likely have a different significance than the first.

Birthdays, Mother's Day and Father's Day, Valentine's Day, the Fourth of July and religious holidays are family gatherings that may remind you of who is missing from around the table, but still lives deeply in your heart. Be gentle with yourself on these days. Plan special things to do and tell others what you want to happen on these days. You may find that sometimes the anticipation and build-up may be worse than the day itself.

There are a number of things you can do as you face these special days:

- Find time alone to think, meditate and/or pray.
- Talk with a support person about how you feel and what you need.
- Treat yourself to something special, dinner out, a sporting event, shopping, a bubble bath or a night in a hotel. Do something for yourself and for each other that will be comforting and will pamper you at the same time.
- Write a letter or poem to your baby. Write in a journal or just on scratch paper.
- Create or buy a special memento to honor your baby.
- Have a special candle that you light whenever you are feeling especially vulnerable and close to the baby. This symbol can become a signal to those around you to tread lightly and share hugs freely.
- Take some time off work if that might be helpful.
- Make a donation in memory of or in honor of your baby to a special charity.
- Alter traditions if the current ones are too painful for you right now.

"Though I have yet to reach my due date, I would like to think that amidst the sadness of the day, I can also reflect on the miracle of life that I had for almost six months inside of me. I hope to smile at least once for the wonderful feeling it was to have been pregnant." Holli

"My hardest part was my due date. I should have a beautiful, live child now. I felt that God was punishing me for what I had done wrong through my life. That's why all this mess happened." Jackie

"It was hard to pretend it was just 'another' day. The mail that day brought a diaper service congratulations coupon. My sister-in-law's baby shower was the day before my due date. I did not go. For Christmas we bought the baby some ornaments and put them on the tree. This helped to make him real and a part of our family." J

"My due date was very hard. I took a long look at what 'should have been,' and had a 'fantasy day' where I played it out the way it should have happened." S.

"My due date is fast approaching and it is very difficult. Every time I see someone very pregnant, and they seem to be coming out of the woodwork, I feel jealous because that's how I'm supposed to look right now." Shelley

"Special days I had thought would be happy are now so hard. I had looked forward to Thanksgiving and Christmas, imagining how wonderful they would be with all the anticipation. Now it will be so painful." Dorothy

"For the rest of our lives, our son's birthday will be special. We will not work on that day. Joe helps in planning that day. One year we had a memorial service by the priest who baptized him; another year we went to the shore for two days. Each year Joe lets go of the appropriate number of helium balloons at Frank's grave. A new Christmas ornament is purchased each year with his name and date on it." Cubby

"I have found it difficult around the time the baby was conceived and the anniversary of his death. It's normal to feel sad around the anniversary dates and holidays. It has been helpful to me to not fight these feelings." Susan

"I remember Amy's and Lisa's first birthday so well. I was scared of it coming; happy for Amy but wondering what it would have been like if her twin sister, Lisa, were there. I also did not know for sure what to do in terms of the guests. Did Grandpa, Grandma and others want to go to Lisa's grave? I decided to ask them, and yes, everyone wanted to do that. We went and cried and prayed together at her grave. Only then could I be happy for Amy on her first birthday." Barb.

Dare we try again for another baby? How long should we wait?

You have been hurt so deeply. You may ask yourself how you could ever risk setting yourself up for such hurt again by attempting another pregnancy. You probably feel vulnerable and worried that if this happened to you once it could happen again. You will never again be able to approach a pregnancy in the same worry-free, trusting way. You now know that the worst can happen. Your innocence is lost. You may look at other people's babies with awe, thinking it was such a miracle that all went right. You may marvel at the perfection of other children and wonder if you will ever be able to experience that joy.

"Our child lives a good life, though there are the painful and frustrating times. We fear that if we ever dare to try again for another baby,

something like this, or worse, may happen. It's a scary thought. I wish there were guarantees." Mark

"After Stacey died I did not think I would ever want to try again. But as the months went on I knew that I did want to try again. After all, the geneticist said there was only a two percent chance of it happening again. So right from the start I found a high risk doctor." Faye

Many people express an intense need to fill the immense void of loss after their child has died or is born with abnormalities. There may be times that you ache to be pregnant again and have a healthy child. Maybe you even think another pregnancy will erase the pain of the loss in this pregnancy. At other times, you may be so fearful or worried that you cannot imagine trying again. Each child and pregnancy is unique and can never be replaced or altered by another pregnancy or baby. The child who has died or lives with special needs can never be replaced, forgotten, or made up for. While you have lost your dreams, and for this you grieve, there comes a time when you must go forward and work on building new dreams. Maybe there are reasons why there can be no more babies. This will be a challenge to deal with, but through good communication and openness you will meet it.

"Another pregnancy looks out of the question. I guess the finality of motherhood is really hitting me hard. This was not fair! I feel cheated. I always wanted four children. But then I can remember, I do have Michael. He was real." Jackie

When is the right time to try again? There really is no answer for this. It must be an individual and personal choice. Be assured that you can make it through no matter when your next pregnancy occurs. If, however, you wish to try to find a time that feels right, then give it some thought, regain your health and talk about it for awhile before you go ahead. You may also want to discuss this with your physician.

Be careful not to rush into another pregnancy too fast, hoping to fill the ache in your arms and make the emptiness go away. It doesn't work quite like that. The pain is still there. Instead, try to find ways to express your grief, your love and to remember this baby. Take it slowly, even if you feel age or circumstances encourage you to hurry. You will probably find that there will be days, and then maybe weeks, when you feel you are beginning to be ready to have the love, hope and strength to go through another pregnancy.

"Some days I cling to my 19-month-old son to reassure myself that I am a competent mother. I remember holding my stomach and our baby

73

girl inside and sobbing because I, the mommy, couldn't change the disorders she was diagnosed as having (Trisomy 18). There was so much pain and guilt knowing I could never kiss away her tears and tell her everything would be all right. This made me doubt my ability to have the strength and courage to try again for another child." Holli

Genetic counseling and other medical discussions might be helpful as you consider another pregnancy. If you need a referral to a genetic counselor, ask your doctor or call your local hospital for information on these professionals who might be in your area. Learning about risks, tests and possible options may be helpful in your decisions about future pregnancies. Although some increased risk might be identified, it often is not as high as you fear.

"We went through genetic counseling afterward looking for answers and yet being afraid of hearing that one of us had caused this to happen to our baby or that the chances were high that it would happen again." Mark

You may decide *not* to risk another pregnancy or be unable to get pregnant again. Maybe this is due to age, previous infertility or pregnancy experiences, the risk of another problem with a subsequent baby, or for other reasons. If this possibly is the case for you, there will be additional grief over the loss of the future babies you will not have. It may be very difficult to end on this note. Communication with your partner, family, clergy and possibly a counselor, will be important over the upcoming months. Be kind to yourself. This will not be an easy time. But have hope and believe that with time and support you will survive and grow.

If you are thinking of trying again, be sure you are doing it for the right reasons. If your baby died, you cannot avoid the grief of your loss, no matter how many subsequent pregnancies you have. Don't try to get pregnant in order to put this one behind you or to strive for a healthy baby. Instead, face your pain, get help, seek support and put off another pregnancy at least until you are feeling healthy and ready to risk your love again. This may be months or it may be longer. Try to give yourself adequate time to recover physically and emotionally. No one can tell you the best or right time for another pregnancy, but don't rush into it unless time is of the essence. Then listen to your inner self about how ready you feel to face this again.

One suggestion that professionals and some parents share is to be aware that if your next pregnancy shares the same general time frame and due date, you may experience constant reminders and additional pain. If you think this might be hard, try to plan your pregnancy for a different time of year. However, if you find yourself pregnant with a similar time frame, please know that many families have survived this. Your attitude and honesty about the pain and joy you feel will help you immensely.

"I am now, eight months past Jonathon's death, in my third month of a new pregnancy. We have only told family at this point and have received mixed reactions. Some are very happy for us and supportive. Others have implied that we should have left it alone. Why risk possibly having to go through it again? We haven't told our three children. I don't want them to worry. I'm doing enough of that for all of us. And how I've changed! Yes, I will have an amnio this time and I will not wear blinders about the possibilities of birth defects. I feel very old this time, not any wiser, just more enlightened. I still think about Jonathon a lot in this pregnancy. While it fills me with happiness, it also makes me miss him even more." E.

My partner and I disagree about having another baby.

Disagreement between partners about another baby happens more than you could imagine. Often dad may not want to see his partner go through this again. The pain and fear may be too great for one partner. Or one feels the risks are too high and far outweigh the need or desire to have another baby. Unfortunately, there is no middle ground on this decision, except possibly adoption. Either you try to have another child or you do not. Of course, there is no guarantee that because you try for one you will get pregnant. This disagreement can cause considerable conflict in a relationship. Even sexual problems can occur, since sex is tied to making a baby. This is common and should be discussed. Sometimes, the best approach is to "decide not to decide" for awhile. If possible, put the decision on hold for six months or so. Agree on an amount of time in which to wait until you make your decision. Then spend that time healing yourselves emotionally and physically. Do not dwell on your differences; it can eat away at your entire relationship. Instead, try to strengthen and build your relationship. You have both suffered and need each other's support. When you feel ready or at the end of the agreed upon time, sit down and discuss this issue again. If at this point, or at any other time in the previous or subsequent months, you find yourselves going nowhere and the stress is very intense, you may want to seek out a third party, such as a counselor. They are trained to help mediate difficult decisions.

AFTER TIME HAS PASSED

Over time, and with patience and hard work, you will find that you have survived. Of course, good support, open communication and using good coping skills will aid you in your healing. When you have begun to heal there will be days when you may want to look back, reliving and retelling what happened. Make room for the tears to still flow, the anger, sadness and other feelings to be there. You will never forget what has happened, whether your child lives or has died. Reminders of the loss of your dreams and hopes may overcome you on some days and may be very distant on others. You will probably experience many more good days and find you can look to the future with hope.

Be positive, trust your faith and believe that you *are* healing. Continue to go forward, with occasional glances back. You will likely gain wisdom, strength and comfort. Remember the memories need not be all hard and sad, but rather a part of the growth that comes from this experience and your baby and the love you hold in your heart.

"I am surprised at how acute and painful my grief still feels three months later. I have had three miscarriages in the past and was much more able to move on with my life. Tears come so easily and so frequently. It feels like no one understands." Dorothy

"Though our baby died shortly after birth, I'm glad we let it happen the way it did. We were able to experience the pain and joy of the last few months of pregnancy. We held her when she died, we loved her deeply when she lived. What more could we do? Now our challenge is to go on, without her in our arms, but forever in our hearts." M.

"Even though our baby is blind and has other problems, we are thankful for his life. Most days are good, though not always. We take it a day at a time. It is harder to control things now and we can't plan too far in advance, but overall we would do this over if given the choice. Having a supportive and loving family really helps us cope." Nancy

"We made the best out of a tough situation. I have few regrets, lots of support and tons of positives to hold on to. The pictures, mementos and memories of the time with our baby give us comfort, and we are so thankful for them. I work on having a positive attitude because I

strongly feel that we can become what we strive for and believe. I seek acceptance, peace and happiness. I know it is coming." Jan

"Birthdays and holidays are especially poignant as they are painful reminders of the sacrifice the babies made so that Tayna and Tammy could live. We feel blessed and happy most days. There are times when we feel the closeness of all four of our babies and the tears of love, sadness and joy flow freely." Jeanne

The sight of other pregnant mothers and parents of young children, especially those of similar ages as yours, may be very painful. You may find commercials, the baby section of the grocery store, magazine ads, marketing pieces that come to your home, baptisms, births and showers difficult and even painful. They probably remind you of your love for your baby and how things have changed. If you feel like avoiding these situations then do avoid them. The daily struggles may not be easy, so be strong about seeking the support you need. As you heal from the inside out you will gradually be able to see the joy in these situations again.

"I am confronted with healthy babies and pregnant women even at work. It has been very painful at times." Joette

"I still miss my baby. The pain can be very raw at times. But my motherly love helps me keep the good memories of her alive as I slowly heal." D.

Keep moving and growing as you work toward healing. Remember that you will always love your baby and the dream of what your baby could have been and done. Whether your baby lives a challenged life or has died, seek support, do what you need to do, live each day fully, cherish the memories, and slowly release the dreams you once held while you create new dreams.

The pain never goes away completely. It can get easier to bear over time. Grieve deeply and completely and be gentle with yourself as you travel toward new beginnings.

It is a risk to attempt new beginnings.
Yet, the greater risk is for you to risk nothing.
For there will be no further possibilities
of learning and changing,
of traveling upon the journey of life.
You were strong to hold on.
You will be stronger to go forward to new beginnings.

Earl Grollman, from his book, *Time Remembered,* 1987

Hope...Time...Love...Healing

Tomorrow will come. The pain will ease. But you will always love your precious child. It takes hope and time and love for the healing to take place.
Remember along the way to accept, but never forget.

Empty Arms, 1990

APPENDIX

National Resources

SUPPORT AND INFORMATION

Abiding Hearts, P.O. Box 5245, Bozeman, MT 59717 (406) 587-7421
A support system for parents continuing pregnancy after prenatal diagnosis of fatal, or non-fatal, birth defects.

Centering Corporation 1531 N. Saddle Creek Rd., Omaha, NE 68104-5064 (402) 553-1200
Offers hundreds of books and booklets on grief, dying, saying goodbye and exceptional children and situations. Catalog available.

Compassionate Friends P.O. Box 3696, Oak Brook, IL 60522-3696 (708) 990-0010
A self-help organization for bereaved parents that has support group chapters worldwide, a newsletter, literature and other resources for families who have had a child of any age die from any cause.

A Place To Remember, Suite 110, 1885 University Ave., St. Paul, MN 55104 (612) 645-7045
Mail order offering birth/death announcement and sympathy cards, baby memory box/book, and other books and booklets for the family and careproviders.

M.O.S.T. (Mothers of Supertwins), P.O. Box 951, Brentwood, NY 11717 (516) 434-6678
National support network for families who are expecting or are already parents of triplets or more. Offers newsletter, patient education, expectant and new parent packages.

Our Newsletter (CLIMB, Inc.) P.O. Box 1064, Palmer, AK 99645 (907) 746-6123
A support network by and for parents who have experienced the death at birth, or in infancy of one, both or all of their children during a multiple pregnancy.

Parent Care 9041 Colgate St., Indianapolis, IN 46268-1210 (317) 872-9913
Parents and professionals dedicated to improving the newborn intensive care experience and future for babies, families and caregivers. Newsletter, literature, referrals to groups and annaul national conference.

Pen Parents, Inc. P.O. Box 8738, Reno, NV 89507-8738 (702) 826-7332
A correspondence network for parents who have suffered through termination, pregnancy loss or the death of a child. Two newsletters: **"P.A.I.L.S of Hope"** Pregnancy & Parenting After Infertility/Loss Support and **"A Heartbreaking Choice,"** for parents who have interrupted their pregnancies.

79

The Triplet Connection, P.O. Box 99571, Stockton, CA 95209
(209) 474-0885
Provides vital information, encouragement, information, resources and networking for families expecting or who already have larger multiples. A good resource for professionals also. Offers a newsletter and packets of extensive information.

SHARE St. Joseph's Health Center, 300 First Capitol Dr, St. Charles, MO 63301
(800) 821-6819
Offers support to families who have had a miscarriage, stillbirth or infant death, including pregnancy termination. Provides a newsletter, network of worldwide support groups, literature and referrals.

Wintergreen Press, 3630 Eileen Street, Maple Plain, MN 55359
(612) 476-1303
Mail order catalog offers books, cards, booklets, videos and slides on infant loss and bereavement.

ADOPTION

National Adoption Center 1500 Walnut St., Suite 701, Philadelphia, PA 19102 (800) 862-3678
Information and referral service for special needs adoption. Offers state resource lists of adoption agencies, parent and advocacy groups. The Adoption Exchange matches families looking to adopt children with special needs.

GENETICS AND SPECIAL NEEDS

Alliance of Genetic Support Groups 35 Wisconsin Circle, Suite 440, Chevy Chase, MD 20815 (800) 336-4363 or (301) 652-5553
Provides educational materials and referrals to consumers regarding most birth defects and genetic disorders. Referrals to parents, genetics professionals, support groups and organizations.

Cystic Fibrosis Foundation 6931 Arlington Rd., Suite 200, Bethesda, MD 20814 (800) 344-4823 or (301) 951-4422
Offers information and referrals to local chapters, support groups, medical information and newsletter.

March of Dimes Birth Defects Foundation 1275 Mamaroneck Ave., White Plains, NY 10605 (914) 428-7100
Offers information, referrals and education on many prenatal, pregnancy and child related issues with a focus on healthy mothers and healthy babies.

National Down Syndrome Congress 1605 Chantilly Dr., Suite 250, Atlanta, GA 30324 (800) 232-6372 (NDSC)
Offers support, literature and education on Down Syndrome.

National Information Center For Children & Youth With Handicaps Box 1492, Washington, DC 20013 (800) 999-5599 TT (703) 893-8614
Provides information and referrals for children with disabilities, early intervention, education, support and literature.

NORD (National Organization of Rare Disorders) P.O. Box 8923, New Fairfield, CT 06812-1783 (203) 746-6518
Provides information on rare diseases, a referral network of parents and a data base of information and educational materials.

National Society of Genetic Counselors, Inc. 233 Canterbury Lane, Wallingford, PA 19086
Most practicing genetic counselors are members of NSGC. Makes referrals to genetic counselors and has patient educational materials on genetic counseling and some common disorders. Only accepts requests for information in writing.

SOFT (Support Organization for Trisomy 18, 13, and related disorders) 21 Ryers Ave., Cheltenham, PA 19012 (215) 663-9652
Offers newsletter and referrals to support groups and parents of trisomic children.

Spina Bifida Association of America 4590 MacAurthur Blvd. NW, Suite 250, Washington DC 20007 (800) 621-3141 or (202) 944-3285
Offers information, newsletter, literature, advocacy, research and referrals to local groups and agencies.

POST-ABORTION SUPPORT

Open Arms, P.O. Box 1056, Columbia, MO 65205 (314) 449-7672
A Christian post abortion ministry dedicated to help anyone who is suffering after an abortion or pregnancy termination.

PACE, Care Net, a ministry of the Christian Action Counsel, 101 West Broad St., Suite 500, Falls Church, VA 22046 (703) 237-2100
Offers referrals to local pregnancy care centers who provide counseling and Bible study.

Works Cited

Granat, Diane. January 1991. "Precious Lives, Painful Choices." *The Washingtonian.*
Green, Rose. 1992. "Letter to a Genetic Counselor." *Journal of Genetic Counseling*, vol. 1, no. 1, 1: 55-70.
Helmstetter, Shad. 1988. *Choices.* Pocket Books.
Ilse, Sherokee. 1982-1990. *Empty Arms: Coping with Miscarriage, Stillbirth and Infant Death.* Minneapolis: Wintergreen Press.
Wheeler, David D. 1980. *Practical Guide for Making Decisions.* Free Press.

BIBLIOGRAPHY
BOOKS AND BOOKLETS

Books, groups or resources may be biased and may or may not be helpful to you. Screen carefully and know that it's okay to use what feels right and leave the rest.

The Anguish of Loss, Julie Fritsch with Sherokee Ilse, Wintergreen Press, 1988. A sensitive photographic resource of sculptures and prose that "allows the reader to move beyond the intellectual concepts of bereavement and enter into the loss experience: the raw, naked anguish of those long, lonely months."

Anna, A Daughter's Life, William Loizeaux, Arcade Publishing, NY, 1993. Born with a number of birth defects known as VATER syndrome, Anna's chances for survival were uncertain. Each day was a gift, and each moment was precious. Much of her brief life was spent in hospital nurseries and operating rooms, yet her father shares how Anna transformed her parents' lives. This stunningly beautiful record of a father's grief becomes an act of celebration.

The Baby Doctors: Probing the Limits of Fetal Medicine, Gina Kolata, Delcorte Press, 1990. A look at the work that doctors are doing on babies *in utero* who have problems such as diaphragmatic hernia and bladder obstructions. Also discusses selective reduction of multiple pregnancies. This book probes the limits of high tech, as new treatments are explored in reproductive medicine and fetal diagnosis and therapy.

Beyond Prenatal Choice, Genetic Counselors, Centering Corporation. A small booklet that offers support to the family choosing an abortion. Good information and recognition of feelings.

Bittersweet Baby, A family meets the challenge of a child with disabilities, Jolie Kanat, Compcare, 1987. A personal journey of a family parenting their baby who has Down syndrome. Addresses grief, guilt, pain, sorrow, hope and recovery.

Bittersweet...hellogoodbye, Sr. Jane Marie Lamb, editor, National SHARE. A large compilation of service ideas, poems, prose, songs to help in planning a memorial service/funeral for a baby.

Children with Disabilities: A Medical Primer, Mark Batshaw, M.D. and Yvonne Perret, M.A., MSW, Brookes Publishing, 1992. An excellent sourcebook that discusses questions, hopes, concerns, ethical dilemmas, explanations of disabilites, causes, intervention and treatment strategies and extensive resources for mental, emotional, learning and physical disabilities. A good book to have early in the process.

Coping with Infant or Fetal Loss: The couple's healing process, Kathleen Gilbert, Ph.D. and Laura Smart, Ph.D., Brunner/Mazel Publishers, 1992. A book from which to gather information and inspiration as partners search for a way to live with their loss and move on. It is realistic and hopeful.

Difficult Decisions, Centering Corporation, 1990. A good section on the actual hospital experience, feelings and the weeks that follow a pregnancy termination. Includes many individual's stories and quotes.

Down Syndrome, Now What Do I Do? Anne and Andrew Squires, Indian Orchard Publishing, 1990. A resource book of advice, questions and answers, organizations, books and other helpful information for families.

Empty Arms: Coping with Miscarriage, Stillbirth and Infant Death, Sherokee Ilse, Wintergreen Press, 1982/1990. Sensitively guides families through the first moments, the options and decisions, the early days and the healing process. Also includes other types of losses that relate to babies: adoption, termination, and SIDS. For families and professionals.

Empty Cradle, Broken Heart, Deborah Davis, Fulcrum Publishing, 1991. A comprehensive and sensitive look at the grief and healing of families after miscarriage, stillbirth and infant death. For families and professionals.

For Better or Worse, For Couples Whose Child Has Died, Maribeth Wilder Doerr, Centering Corp, 1992. An easy to read book which deals with marriage and relationships after a child dies.

Having Your Baby When Others Say No! Overcoming the Fears about Having Your Baby, Madeline Pecora Nugent, Avery Publishing Group, NY, 1991. A sensitive guide to support women who choose to continue their pregnancy amidst crisis, health problems and fear. Many true-life stories of women who were told or encouraged to end their pregnancies but who instead chose to deliver them and in some cases give the baby up for adoption. Extensive resource section deals with financial and legal assistance.

Helping Women Recover From Abortion, Nancy Michels, Bethany House, 1988. Christian based ideas on how to deal with guilt, emotional pain and emptiness following abortion. Includes chapters on grief, denial, guilt, anger, forgiveness, scripture and nine steps for personal growth.

Helping Your Exceptional Baby: A Practical and Honest Approach to Raising a Mentally Handicapped Baby, Cliff Cunningham and Patricia Sloper, Pantheon, 1981. Questions and answers, practical advice and good resources.

Loving and Letting Go, Deborah L. Davis, Ph.D., Centering Corporation, 1993. This book about letting go and allowing nature to take its course is for parents who want to turn away from aggressive medical intervention for their critically ill newborn.

Meditations for Bereaved Parents, Judy Osgood, Gilgal Publications, P.O. Box 3386, Sunriver, OR 97707, 1983. Spiritual and healing meditations written by the bereaved for the bereaved.

A Mother's Dilemma: A spiritual search for meaning following pregnancy interruption after prenatal diagnosis, Wendy Lyon with Molly Minnick, Pinneapple Press, P.O. Box 56, Mullett Lake, MI 49761, 1993. This book is about forgiveness—forgiveness of self, of each other, of God and of due process.

Post-Abortion Trauma, Jeanette Vought, Zondervan, 1991. Women and men openly share their stories after having an abortion. Addresses the church's response, support networks and outlines a nine-step recovery precess.

Precious Lives, Painful Choices: A prenatal decision-making guide, Sherokee Ilse, Wintergreen Press, 1993. A comprehensive, balanced guide for families in the throes of decision making when they learn their unborn child has problems. Addresses issues for continuing and terminating the pregnancy, as well as support for surviving the days and months that follow.

Pregnancy Heartbreak: Unfulfilled Promises, by parents who have either terminated or continued their pregnancies following prenatal diagnosis. A short booklet for use in the beginning days and while in the hospital. Abbott Northwestern Hospital, 800 E. 28th St. & Chicago Ave., Minneapolis, MN 55407-3799.

Prenatal Tests, What They Are, Their Benefits and Risks and How to Decide Whether to Have Them or Not, Robin Blatt, Vintage Books, 1988. What are they and what are the risks/benefits of prenatal tests? Explores the pros and cons of screening tests and encourages informed decision-making.

Remembering with Love, Elizabeth Levang and Sherokee Ilse, Deaconess Press, 1992. An affirming gift for those grieving the loss of a loved one. This daily inspirational guide offers compassion, comfort, support and guidance as it teaches about grief, healing and hope.

The Rights of Patients, George J. Annas, JD, MPH, 1992. A completely revised and updated second edition of the classic book which clearly spells out patients' rights. The question and answer format helps patients be informed about such issues as their right to refuse treatment, how to use medical and law libraries and finding other resources.

Searching for the Stork: One Couple's Struggle to Start a Family, Marion Lee Wasserman, New American Library, NY, 1990. A powerful account of a couple's struggle with multiple pregnancy loss and genetic disease, molar pregnancy and pregnancy termination. This personal story shares the heartache and trauma in a realistic way.

The Self-Help Sourcebook: Finding and Forming Mutual Aid Self-Help Groups, found in libraries and can be ordered from: The New Jersey Self-Help Clearinghouse, St. Clare's Riverside Medical Center, Pocono Rd., Denville, NJ 07834, 201-625-9565. Gives information on forming self-help groups and lists over 1,000 self-help groups in the U.S. Includes information on groups dealing with children with special needs or who are terminally ill, infant death, rare disorders and genetic disorders.

A Silent Sorrow, Pregnancy Loss, Guidance and Support for You and Your Family, Ingrid Kohn, MSW and Perry-Lynn Moffitt, Dell , 1993. Covers the many aspects of miscarriage, stillbirth and infant death including the couple's relationships, siblings and faith issues. Chapter 8 deals specifically with The Burden of Choice.

The Special Child: A Source Book for Parents of Children with Developmental Disabilities, Siegfried Pueschel and James Bernier, Paul H. Brooks, 1988. Full of information, books, organizations and other resources.

Still to be Born, Pat Schwiebert, RN, & Paul Kirk, MD, Perinatal Loss, 2116 NE 18th Ave, Portland, OR 97212. For the couple still grieving and longing for another baby, but afraid of being hurt again by another loss

The Tentative Pregnancy: Prenatal Diagnosis and the Future of Motherhood, B.K. Rothman, Penguin Books, 1986. Critically examines the impact of prenatal diagnosis, especially amniocentesis on childbearing and bonding.

Tilly, Frank Perriti, Cross Ways Books, 1988. A deeply moving novel of life, love, abortion, and Christ's forgiveness that is both gentle and healing.

A Time to Decide, A Time to Heal, Molly Minnick, MSW, editor, Pineapple Press, 1990. An 82-page booklet that offers assistance especially for those who have or might interrupt a pregnancy. Support for the days and months ahead and future pregnancies.

When Bad Things Happen to Good People, Rabbi Harold Kushner, Simon & Schuster, 1981. This book takes the view that God "allows" the world to take its course and hurts for you, but is there for comfort and support when circumstances bring about bad things. The author speaks from personal experience as his son suffered and died.

When Hello Means Goodbye, Pat Schwiebert and Paul Kirk, Perinatal Loss, 1977. A booklet to aid grieving families in the early days after a pregnancy or infant loss.

When Pregnancy Fails, Susan Borg and Judith Lasker, Bantam, 1981/1989. A thorough look at pregnancy loss and infant death incorporating fathers, couples, singles, other family members, faith and spiritual issues, what next, and much more. Chapter 4 deals exclusively with Prenatal Diagnosis and the Unwanted Abortion.

When Pregnancy Isn't Perfect: A Layperson's Guide to Complications in Pregnancy, Laurie Rich, 1991. By a mother who went through a high risk pregnancy, this book reflects medical, emotional and psychological aspects and intrauterine growth retardation, infections, multiple pregnancy complications, pregnancy loss, and bedrest.

Which Test for My Unborn Baby? Lachlan de Crespigny and Rhonda Dredge, 1991. Offers information on prenatal testing, giving a clear outline of the techniques available and the main ones in use.

Yesterday, I Dreamed of Dreams, compiled by Molly Minnick, Pinneapple Press, 1991. Poems, letters and memorials by parents for loved babies who were aborted after a fetal abnormality was diagnosed.

Your Down's Syndrome Child, Everything Today's Parents Need to Know About Raising Their Special Child, Eunice McClurg, Doubleday, 1986. A personal and compassionate handbook that presents specific situations and concerns likely to occur during the child's development; medical information and research information.

BOOKS FOR CHILDREN

Explaining Death to Children, edited by Rabbi Earl Grollman, Beacon Press, 1967. Excellent collection of articles for parents and professionals to help children. Extensive bibliography.

The Fall of Freddie the Leaf, Leo Bascalgia, Charles Slack Publisher, 1982. Through the beauty of nature, this book presents life as a natural cycle. Freddie and

Daniel talk about life, their purpose, that everything dies and that "we all fear what we don't know."

How Do We Tell The Children? Dan Schaefer and C. Lyons, Newmarket, 1986. Valuable book for parents that offers guidance and information to help families communicate about death.

Lifetimes, The beautiful way to explain death to children, Mellonie and Ingpen. Describes the life cycles, beginnings and endings, with plants, animals and people. Lovely illustrations.

No New Baby: For Boys and Girls Whose Expected Sibling Dies, N. Hagley, Centering Corporation, 1985. A story for children whose baby brother or sister dies in pregnancy or shortly afterrwards. Deals with a child's guilt and sadness.

Tell Me, Papa: A family book for children's questions about death and funerals, Joy and Marv Johnson, Centering Corporation, 1984. Short, readable and addresses many issues children experience when grieving a loved one.

The Tenth Good Thing About Barney, Judith Viorst. A provocative book with good illustrations, about the death and burial of a pet cat.

Thumpy's Story, Nancy Dodge and Sr. Jane Marie Lamb, SHARE. Thumpy, a rabbit, tells of his grief when his sister Bun unexpectedly dies. Beautiful artwork.

ARTICLES, MAGAZINES, REFERENCE BOOKS

Bereavement Magazine, 8133 Telegraph Drive, Colorado Springs, CO 80920, (719)-282-1948. A magazine of hope and healing written by and for bereaved families. Covers all types of grief, full of heart-wrenching stories of hope, pain and healing. This is a support group in print.

Encyclopedia of Associations, Gale Research. Available in most public libraries. A comprehensive book of local, state and national associations and organizations that deal with many problems. Phone numbers and addresses included.

Exceptional Parent Magazine, 1170 Commonwealth Ave., Boston, MA 02134, (617) 730-5800. Once a year this monthly magazine has resource listings for families who have exceptional children including disabilities. Local libraries may have back issues.

Letter to a Genetic Counselor, Rose Green, **Journal of Genetic Counseling,** Vol. 1, No. 1, 1992, pp 55-70. Reflections of a woman who terminated her pregnancy after abnormal amniocentesis results.

Precious Lives, Painful Choices, Diane Granat, **The Washingtonian,** January 1991. Thorough article sharing personal stories and medical facts.

XYLO: A True Story, Rayna Rapp, **Test Tube Women,** edited by Adritti, Klein and Minden , Pandora Press, 1984. Personal account of a woman who learned through amniocentesis that her child had Down syndrome, then terminated the pregnancy.

INDEX

The Anguish of Loss
Julie Fritsch with Sherokee Ilse

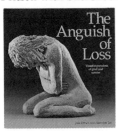

A unique and poignant photographic account of a mother's anguish, pain and movement through grief. These beautiful sculptures and accompanying prose portray the grieving and healing process like no other book.
Book $14.95 Slide/cassette $175

Empty Arms
Sherokee Ilse

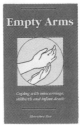

A sensitive guide given to thousands of families each year to aid during the time of their infant loss or miscarriage. Offers guidance, comfort and hope for grieving parents and their families. An extensive bibliography and resource list.
Book $9.95 Bulk rate Video $75
Spanish Version Available.

Miscarriage:A Shattered Dream
Sherokee Ilse and Linda Hammer Burns

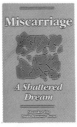

This 68-page resource offers support and guidance for those experiencing a miscarriage or for those who care for them. Sensitive discussion of topics such as: emotional responses, medical, coping skills and memorial suggestions. Extensive resource section.
$9.95 Bulk rate available

Remembering With Love
Elizabeth Levang and Sherokee Ilse

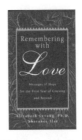

An affirming gift for those grieving the loss of a loved one. Offers comfort, compassion and guidance. Over 300 short passages offer encouragement and information on the normal grieving process, how to cope and have hope.

$11.95

Write for the full catalog which also features many booklets and A-V materials.